BLOOD PRESSURE MANAGEMENT
in Primary Care

Terry McCormack

MBBS DRCOG MRCA

MAGISTER CONSULTING LTD

BLOOD PRESSURE MANAGEMENT IN PRIMARY CARE

Terry McCormack MBBS DRCOG MRCA

Published in the UK by
Magister Consulting Ltd
The Old Rectory
St. Mary's Road
Stone
Dartford
Kent DA9 9AS

Copyright © 2006 Magister Consulting Ltd
Printed in the UK by Hartley Reproductions Ltd, Greenhithe, Kent

ISBN 1 873839 69 3

616.132 0BP

Foreword

Hypertension is diagnosed frequently in primary care and its clinical management represents an important component of the daily work of primary care physicians. The evidence base underpinning recommendations for the treatment of hypertension is the most substantial in medicine. However, new trials continue to emerge and the results of these trials are under constant evaluation. This has led to frequent updates in clinical guidelines from the British Hypertension Society (BHS) and the National Institute of Clinical Excellence (NICE). Amidst these official outputs, there has been much seemingly conflicting information about the special benefits of different drug therapies in the medical and lay press. This presents an enormous challenge to primary care physicians who have to evaluate this information and make decisions about the best treatment options for their patients.

In this book, Terry McCormack has produced an excellent and very readable practical guide for physicians about the assessment and treatment of patients with hypertension. It has been a formidable challenge to review information from many sources and generate such a concise and yet comprehensive review of the key issues facing physicians treating hypertension in primary care. This book is highly topical and covers important emerging issues such as the use of cardiovascular risk assessment to guide treatment decisions, when to use adjunctive therapies such as statins and aspirin, and the interpretation of estimated glomerular filtration rate (eGFR) in clinical practice. This information is put into context alongside the very recent review of the pharmacological treatment of hypertension by the BHS and NICE.

The style of the author is refreshing and very practical, and this book will be an invaluable resource for all primary care physicians, GPs with a special interest, nurse practitioners with an interest in hypertension and pharmacists. Terry McCormack is to be congratulated for producing a user-friendly little gem of a book that promises to be a popular education manual for the practising physician.

Bryan Williams MD FRCP FAHA

Professor of Medicine, Department of Cardiovascular Sciences,
University of Leicester School of Medicine, UK

Contents

Contents

Introduction

This book is intended as an easy-to-read, 'how-to-do-it' guide for primary care doctors and nurses running hypertension clinics. Because it is written by a GP, it should reflect the issues pertinent to hypertension management in primary care and be realistic in terms of what can be done. My knowledge on this subject comes not only from practical experience but also from listening to and talking with various people involved in hypertension, both the experts and other 'coalface workers' like myself. As in any book there is much personal reflection and therefore much of this is my interpretation of the facts. While the evidence is extremely important, it is how you use that evidence that is paramount. I would hope to help the reader to make their own mind up about where they stand in hypertension management. This is particularly vital in writing local guidelines, and I use the protocols of my own practice in this book as examples.

One question we should all ask ourselves is 'What is my bias'? Putting it another way, am I trying to prove that the patient has high blood pressure or prove they have not? Generally it is in our nature to be conservative and wish the patient well - in other words, to try to prove there is no problem. The advantage there is that we avoid unnecessary treatment. But, equally, are we therefore depriving the patient of the advantages of treatment? Ideally we should be neutral observers, and the only way to achieve this is to set some rules and then live with them - hence the need for protocols, whether we like them or not!

We are all aware of the 'rule of halves': half the patients are not diagnosed, half of those who are diagnosed are not treated and, of the ones treated, half are not controlled. The new General Medical Services (nGMS) Contract has changed this quite markedly in that a higher proportion are now being diagnosed and treated and between 60% and 70% are controlled. This is a remarkable achievement and might make the UK a leader in the implementation of good practice. Therefore, my book might be pushing at an opening door. However, wherever you are coming from, you should learn something from this book.

x

Chapter 1

What is hypertension?

Learning objectives

After reading this chapter you should have a better understanding of some of the concepts of how we define high blood pressure as well as some of the myths and misconceptions. We will examine the causes of primary and secondary hypertension and factors related to diagnosis. In particular we will look at the subject in terms of providing an explanation of the condition to the patient. The diagnostic criteria will be related to the current guidelines and government targets.

Key words:

Epidemiologists

Global risk assessment

Dietary salt load

Renin-angiotensin-aldosterone system (RAAS)

Patient explanation

What is hypertension?

So what is hypertension? Is it a disease or just a measurement description? When do we go from being normal to abnormal and how did the physicians who described this condition decide the cut-off points? Why do we get the feeling that the goalposts keep moving and is there any justification for the cynical view that hypertension is over-hyped?

Synonyms of the prefix 'hyper' include tense, nervous, excited, jumpy, anxious, twitchy, edgy and jittery. The suffix 'tension' could be replaced by pressure, worry, nervousness, anxiety, stress, strain or apprehension. Twitchy nervousness or jittery apprehension could certainly describe the patient's reaction to the news that something is wrong with them, especially if, as is usually the case, they are asymptomatic. Of course the intention is that the word 'hypertension' means 'higher than normal pressure', but this is all Greek as far as the patient is concerned. Patients frequently ask what is hypertension, what do the two different numbers mean and the age-old 'why me'? It is important that we can at least try to answer these questions.

The invention of the mercury sphygmomanometer and the realisation that we could use it to measure blood pressure started the process off. In the early 20th Century physicians such as Korotkoff defined the art and science of what the various sounds in the brachial artery meant and how they could be used to estimate both systolic and diastolic blood pressures. The equipment designers improved the accuracy of the apparatus sufficiently for it to come into everyday use and, hey presto, we had a 'must-have' device on every doctor's desk. Herein lies one of the factors that created the importance of blood pressure measurement: availability. Here was a relatively simple, non-invasive and repeatable clinical measurement that calculated a parameter of the cardiovascular system.

Low blood pressure is of course important in terms of evaluating the shocked or compromised patient, and this was probably the first use of the measurement. Then, in the early days of recognising that high pressure was dangerous, it was the people with very high systolic figures, such as those above 250 mmHg, who were felt to be of significance to doctors as they could relate this to associated signs such as retinal changes and concomitant disease such as renal failure. They could also perceive how it might lead to an early death.

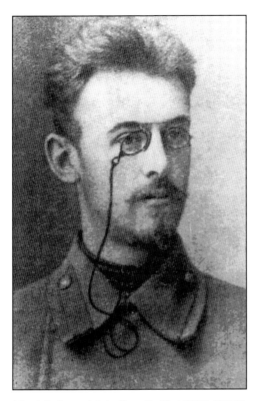

Nicolai Sergeivich Korotkoff (1874-1920)
With kind permission of the Russian Military Medical Academy, Saint Petersburg, Russia

The more common hypertensive condition, one now more significant in terms of the sheer numbers we need to treat, is moderately raised blood pressure. The importance of this aspect of hypertension was realised much later and came from the study of large populations rather than individuals. It was through studies funded by actuaries and insurance companies that we came to understand the importance of moderate rises in blood pressure in 1939.[1] The epidemiologists discovered the relationship between moderate rises and increased mortality. At the time this finding may have caused a bigger stir among insurance actuaries than the medical profession. The fact that moderately higher blood pressure caused disease in no way meant that reducing the pressure would have any beneficial effect. The first evidence that this view needed to change arose only in the late 1960s and into the 1970s with large-scale epidemiological trials such as the Medical Research Council (MRC) Trial.[2]

Having established the fact that not just severe hypertension was relevant, the next question was 'at what cut-off point does normal become abnormal'? In essence this became a committee decision, based on epidemiological and economic evidence, but nonetheless an arbitrary figure was set at the point where it was felt that treatment was more beneficial than harmful. Hence, as newer treatments emerged with fewer side effects, and further evidence of benefits was revealed, the goalposts moved.

If we measure the diastolic and systolic blood pressures of any population then we will derive two sets of normal distribution curves. The majority of people will be in the middle and the outliers will be abnormal. In the case of blood pressure the perception is that those at the upper limit are the people with the problems.

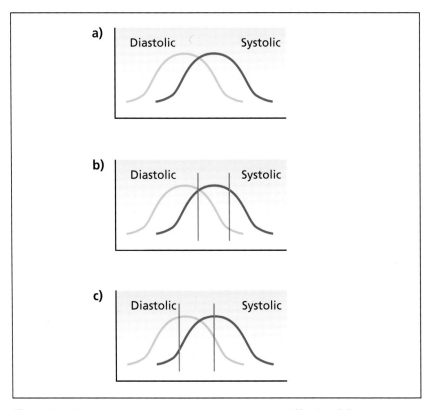

Figure 1.1 Where do you set your blood pressure cut-off points? Do you set them high (b)? Or low (c)?

Do you have graduated lines or a total winners and losers cut-off point? The problem with the arbitrary cut-off is that those close to the line become difficult in terms of their inclusion or exclusion. If the systolic cut-off is 160 mmHg, then how can you say someone has a problem at that exact measurement but is okay at 159 mmHg? You cannot. The initial answer to this was to introduce the 'you are okay but we need to keep a close eye on you in future' attitude. That has now been replaced with the 'you would have been okay but for the other problems you have' attitude or, in other words, global risk assessment. The advent of risk tables that continually relate your blood pressure against various other risk factors such as age, sex, smoking status and cholesterol is an immensely important step forward, but more of that in *Chapter 7*.

Looking back at the two normal distribution curves in *figure 1a*, the most important factor is the make-up of the population studied. Herein lies one of the most popular misconceptions originating in the early days of frequent, routine blood pressure measurement: namely, that it is normal for blood pressure to rise with age. Taking the UK as an example, it was common in the 1970s and 1980s to rely heavily on personal experience to colour one's judgement. It was the experience of all doctors that older patients had higher blood pressure. Hence the myth arose that this was a normal progression of age. It was the emergence of evidence-based medicine in the 1990s that brought home to clinicians something that the epidemiologists had known for sometime, namely that the UK population, like its northern European neighbours, was abnormal. Other populations, especially those in more primitive economic areas, did not have progressively increasing blood pressure with advancing age.

The other question that arose was 'can we do anything about it?' Early studies such as the MRC trial[2] disappointed people because they expected to see a major reduction in events when blood pressure was controlled. While strokes were reduced by about 40% there was a much more tame reduction in coronary heart disease events of only 24%. The main reason for these findings was the fact that treating hypertension in isolation is not the answer. When you combine antihypertensive treatment with other treatment strategies such as lipid therapy you begin to see a better picture, such as that demonstrated in the recent ASCOT trial.[3] Also, if you look at the results in higher-risk patients, you can see benefit even with modest reductions in blood pressure, as illustrated in the World Health Organisation - International Society of Hypertension (WHO-ISH) table below.

Table 1.1 Estimated effects of antihypertensive treatment on cardiovascular risk. Adapted from the WHO-ISH Guidelines[4]		
Absolute risk of a fatal stroke, non-fatal stroke or myocardial infarction over 10 yrs	Number needed to treat (NNT) over 10 years to prevent one event	
	BP reduction 10/5 mmHg	BP reduction 20/10 mmHg
<15%	>40	>20
15-20%	30	20
20-30%	25	17
>30%	<20	<10

So how do we explain to the patient the two numbers: systolic and diastolic? This is how I do it. 'The blood vessels in your body are elastic; they stretch when your heart beats and the highest pressure is achieved when they are fully stretched. That is the top figure. When your heart relaxes the pressure falls, but before it falls to nothing your heart beats again and at the point it starts to beat you reach your bottom figure. It cannot fall to zero, otherwise we would all fall over 60 times a minute!' Simplistic and maybe not entirely accurate, but it does explain the concept and most patients are happy with it.

Why me?

'Why me?' can be more difficult to explain, not least because we do not fully understand the cause of this disorder. High blood pressure is not a disease in itself, but is a condition that increases the risk of disease. Sometimes it is a manifestation of a disease process. For the patient this is a source of great confusion. They feel fine but their doctor keeps piling on more and more pills, sometimes actually making them feel unwell. There is a need to explain that the consequences of not treating patients could be dire and also that side effects of treatment are often temporary. Understanding why treatment is needed and trust in the doctors and nurses providing the treatment is vital to maintain compliance with medication and attendance for follow-up consultations.

A minority of patients, about 5%, have a secondary cause such as renal disease or one of the more exotic causes (as summarised in *box 1.1*), but the vast majority have essential (idiopathic) hypertension. The old joke is that 'idiopathic' does not mean we do not know the cause of a problem but that we know we do not know! We are not totally clueless, however.

Box 1.1

Possible primary factors in hypertension:

- Salt and diet
- Renin (RAAS) over-activity
- Environmental
- Urban stress
- Nitric oxide pathway dysfunction
- Insulin resistance

Secondary causes:

- Renal disease
- Conn's syndrome/primary aldosteronism
- Cushing's syndrome
- Phaeochromocytoma
- Coarctation of aorta
- Iatrogenic
  - steroids
  - NSAIDs
  - contraceptive pill

One current theory is that many hypertensive patients have reached a threshold where their kidneys cannot cope with their dietary salt load. The western diet has an excessive salt content. To ensure homeostasis we have to compensate by increasing salt and water depletion, a natural diuresis. Eventually, as the kidneys age, this fails to work. This explains in part why thiazide diuretics are effective. Afro-Caribbean patients are especially sensitive to salt and, hence, are more responsive to treatment with thiazide diuretics.

Many others may be 'renin hypertensives': people who have an excessively active renin-angiotensin-aldosterone system (RAAS). These people may respond better to the angiotensin-converting enzyme (ACE) inhibitors and angiotensin receptor blockers (ARBs). Typically they are younger, non-black patients. The sympathetic nervous system is part of the same scheme of vascular tone regulation. Specifically it has alpha-1 adrenoceptors responsible for vasoconstriction and beta-2 adrenoceptors involved with vasodilatation. Hence the influence of adrenergic-blocking agents.

There may be some people who have ectopic (non-adrenal) sites of aldosterone production. If this is the case then they have primary aldosteronism, which gives a clinical picture similar to Conn's syndrome but should properly be considered as a hidden secondary group. They will respond to the aldosterone antagonist spironolactone. Conn's syndrome is defined as aldosteronism secondary to an adrenal tumour.

An area still being researched is the role of atrial and brain natriuretic peptides (ANP and BNP), which are released from the heart in response to stretching of the myocardium. They oppose the action of the RAAS system.

Aside from these specific theories there is a mishmash of factors that in combination might explain the phenomenon of hypertension. We know that environmental factors play a part because certain geographical areas have a higher incidence of disease even among immigrants from areas of low incidence. Urban stress and the refined foods we eat may explain this. Insulin resistance is also a factor, and genetics are a possible influence. The biologists point to endothelial-derived releasing factor (EDRF), now more properly referred to as nitric oxide (NO). The results of atherosclerosis also play a part

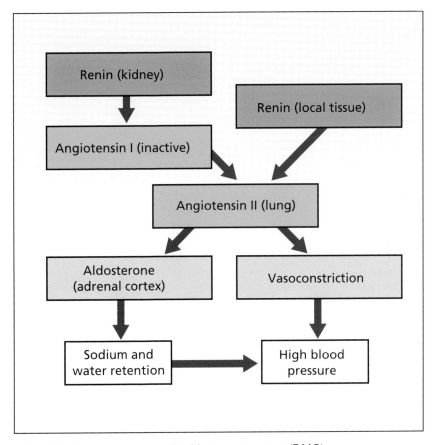

Figure 1.2 The renin-angiotensin-aldosterone system (RAAS)

as the arterial vessel wall loses elasticity and compliance, an age-related factor. The American Heart Association refers to atherosclerotic hypertension as pseudohypertension *(see Chapter 10)*.

Obese patients can have increased blood pressure as a direct result of their weight. They will drop their blood pressure considerably if they lose weight; this reduction is estimated to be in the order of 1 mmHg per kg. Some 'weight-losing' individuals may succeed in removing themselves from the hypertension treatment group and should not then be recorded as being 'hypertensives'.

Another group of 'false' hypertensives are those who go on an alcoholic binge in the 48 hours preceding their blood pressure measurement. During the hangover period the detoxification process causes an overall blood pressure rise due to portal vein congestion, tachycardia and the effect on the RAAS. The alcohol-induced diuresis will gradually reduce this effect. These people should return for measurement following a period of abstinence.

Targets and goalposts

There has been much frustration expressed by those at the coalface of medical practice about the moving goalposts of hypertension targets over the years, but things are settling down. As the epidemiologists accumulate increasingly accurate data, a clearer picture of the situation has evolved. The disbelief regarding the size of the problem is diminishing. We know from the new General Medical Services (nGMS) Contract data that the prevalence of moderate and severe hypertension requiring drug therapy in the entire UK population is 11.3%.

In bygone years many doctors simply gave up on trying to intervene because of the sheer scale of the problem. Government policy now accepts the need for the allocation of resources to tackle the situation and we saw this in both the National Service Framework for Coronary Heart Disease and the nGMS Contract (*table 1.2*[5]). Both of these government initiatives followed the advice of the first Joint British Society Guidelines[6] and the British Hypertension Society Guidelines (*table 1.3*[7]), now in their fourth edition. These establish the need for two types of targets for treatment: optimum targets and the more liberal audit targets by which we can judge success.

The British Guidelines closely match international guidelines such as those of the World Health Organization (WHO) and the Joint National Committee (JNC) Guidelines in the USA.

Before we leave the subject of what hypertension is and my claims that all the previous doubts are being cleared up, let us just throw in a bit of confusion.

Table 1.2 nGMS Contract Quality Outcome Framework Indicators: BP targets (2004 to 2006)[5]

Indicator		Points	Maximum threshold
CHD 6	The percentage of people with coronary heart disease in whom the last blood pressure reading (measured in the last 15 months) is 150/90 mmHg or less	19	70%
Stroke 6	The percentage of people with a history of transient ischaemic attack or stroke in whom the last blood pressure reading (measured in the last 15 months) is 150/90 mmHg or less	5	70%
BP5	The percentage of people with hypertension in whom the last blood pressure (measured in the last 9 months) is 150/90 mmHg or less	57	70%
DM12	The percentage of people with diabetes in whom the last blood pressure is 145/85 mmHg or less	18	60%

Table 1.3 British Hypertension Society Guidelines, IV: classification of BP levels[7]

	Systolic (mmHg)	Diastolic (mmHg)	Treatment
Grade 1 hypertension (mild)	140-159	90-99	Lifestyle (drugs with target organ damage)
Grade 2 hypertension (moderate)	160-179	100-109	Drugs
Grade 3 hypertension (severe)	>180	>110	Drugs

What about the normotensive patients? Do they need treatment too? Trials such as HOPE[8] and PROGRESS[9] have begged the question that there may be no cut-off point where lowering blood pressure is beneficial as long as you pick the right patient. HOPE studied ramipril in normotensive patients with coronary heart disease, reducing mortality by more than 20%, and PROGRESS investigated perindopril in normotensive patients with cerebrovascular disease, reducing recurrence by more than 20%. Furthermore, questions as to the effect of white coat hypertension and the relatively unknown concept of masked hypertension arise, both of which we will tackle later in the book. Nothing is ever straightforward in medicine!

Key points

- Effects of severe hypertension are evident in diseased individuals

- Effects of moderate hypertension are evident in population studies

- Global risk assessment and treatment is more efficient and effective than merely considering single risk factors

References

1. Blood pressure study, 1939. New York: Actuarial Society of America and Association of Life Insurance Medical Directors, 1940

2. Working Party, Medical Research Council. *BMJ* 1992;304:405-412

3. Dahlof B, Sever P, Poulter N et al. *Lancet* 2005;366:895-906

4. 1999 World Health Organization/International Society of Hypertension Guidelines for the Management of Hypertension. *Hypertension* 1999; 17:151-183

5. www.dh.gov.uk/PolicyAndGuidance/OrganisationPolicy/PrimaryCare/PrimaryCareContracting

6. Wood DA, Durrington P, Poulter N et al. *Heart* 1998;80:S1-S29

7. Williams B. Poulter NR. Brown MJ et al. *J Hum Hypertens* 2004;18(3):139-185

8. The Heart Outcomes Prevention Evaluation Study Investigators. *New Engl J Med* 2000;342:145-153

9. PROGRESS Collaborative Group. *Lancet* 2001;358:1033-1041

Chapter 2

Measurement

Learning objectives

Accurate measurement of the patient's blood pressure is vital, but in practice it is often taken erroneously. In this chapter you will learn how to measure blood pressure correctly. We will discuss both the advantages and pitfalls associated with electronic devices. We will consider the future of mercury and aneroid sphygmomanometers. The place of 24-hour monitoring and home measurement of blood pressure will be explored, especially with regard to white coat hypertension.

Key words:

Automated sphygmomanometers

Home measurement

Ambulatory blood pressure

White coat hypertension

Masked hypertension

How to take the blood pressure

If the patient is nervous and the doctor is rushed, there is little chance of an accurate blood pressure measurement being achieved. That the patient is nervous must be taken as the normal situation, even if they do not outwardly feel these nerves or express their fears. Most of our data on blood pressure are derived from such patients in a clinical situation. Therefore our decisions as to what constitutes normal and abnormal readings are based on the clinical or 'office' reading.

Box 2.1

How to measure BP:

- Patient seated for at least 5 minutes, ideally 10
- Arm should be supine and level with the heart
- The patient must be comfortable
- Always use the same arm
- Cuff can be placed over thin clothing
- Use the correct cuff
- Do not undress the patient
- Average of two measurements
- Measurements 1 minute apart, ideally 2 minutes
- Elderly require standing BP also

Every effort must be made to make the patient feel relaxed and rested. Even if they have only just walked from the waiting room to the seat where their measurement is to be made, they cannot be considered to be resting. They must be seated for a minimum of 5 and ideally 10 minutes to achieve the resting state. Their upper arm must be level with their heart and resting on a desk or pillow in a comfortable position. The arm should be supine (palm facing upwards). The cuff must be the correct size and all equipment should have medium and large cuffs readily available. I always put the cuff on as soon as they sit down. This usually stops them from standing up again and causing a delay in achieving a resting state. Try and avoid embarrassing the patient by asking them to undress excessively. If thin clothing is worn on the upper arm, place the cuff over it as this is unlikely to influence the reading, while asking a patient to take off a shirt or blouse could push the blood pressure up considerably.

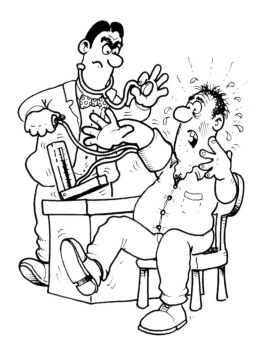

Every effort must be made to make the patient feel relaxed and rested

I usually take one reading immediately. If it is normal then that is quite acceptable. If it were raised I would ignore it completely and now wait 5 or 10 minutes before repeating it. You must wait at least 1 and ideally 2 minutes between measurements to allow the arm to return to its normal resting haemodynamic state. If I am busy, I will still invest that time in waiting, as bringing patients back wastes my time, their time and probably increases anxiety. I can always wander off and do something else or tackle some other issue with the patient that does not require them moving. If at 5 minutes the blood pressure is raised then I must wait another 5 minutes, but at that point I will accept the reading as accurate. At whichever point I decide that I do have an accurate, rested reading, I should wait 1 minute and repeat the test, taking the average of the two readings as the result that will be recorded. If the patient is elderly or in poor general health I will then ask them to stand and take a further measurement after 1 minute to exclude postural hypotension. If a patient does have postural hypotension then the standing blood pressure should be used and recorded as if it is the sitting measurement *(see Chapter 10)*.

Alternatively, if the doctor feels too pressured to make such delayed recordings, they should arrange for the blood pressure to be recorded by someone else, such as a healthcare assistant, who can go to the trouble to wait.

In the assessment phase it is recommended that you record the blood pressure in both arms to see if there is a significant difference and from then onwards use the arm with the highest measurement. However, we always use the left arm in our practice simply because all our desks are that way around! Sometimes practicality will take precedence over pure science.

Which equipment should be used?

Mercury sphygmomanometers

The mercury sphygmomanometer was rumoured to have had its day on safety grounds. However, at the time of writing, the Medicines and Healthcare products Regulatory Authority (MHRA) stated that there are no plans to withdraw mercury sphygmomanometers, although mercury thermometers are likely to be restricted.[1] The main reason for this is that you will continue to need to use mercury devices in patients with arrhythmias. However, you are required to observe health and safety rules on cleaning up mercury spills following breakage, and this can be both inconvenient and expensive. While the equipment itself is accurate it does require 6-monthly column cleaning and calibration. It is also important that the mercury column is kept vertical. Old fold-down-type machines can be inaccurate if the lid holding the column has worn hinges and does not click into a true vertical position.

The person operating the mercury device invariably introduces some inaccuracy. In particular the interpretation of the Korotkoff sounds may vary from person to person. Observer bias is introduced by virtue of whether the clinician wants a high or a low figure and, of course, we can always cheat if we wish to. The greatest bias is in rounding up and down. A scatter diagram is included below *(figure 2.1)*, showing all the readings in my own practice before and after the introduction of automatic sphygmomanometers. While we had a practice policy of recording blood pressure to 2 mmHg you can see from the scattergram that the most common readings were divisible by 10 mmHg and that this bias disappeared when the new equipment came into use.

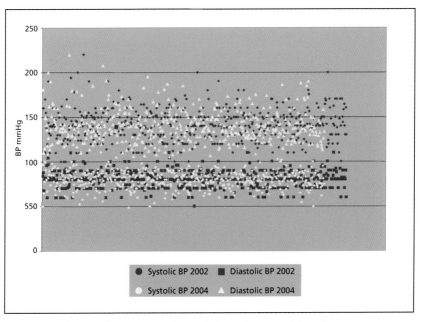

Figure 2.1 Scatter diagram showing variability in manual blood pressure measurement in diabetic patients, 2002 to 2004

Aneroid sphygmomanometers

The alternatives to mercury devices are automatic or manual aneroid sphyg-momanometers. The former are now both affordable and reliable. The latter still permit observer bias, but many clinics may prefer them to mercury devices for those patients in whom automatic sphygmomanometers do not work - ie patients with very high blood pressure or arrhythmias such as atrial fibrillation. Aneroid sphygmomanometers rely on a bellow and spring device that gradually wears out, so they become progressively less accurate with continued use. They are also susceptible to damage if dropped, and this may result in them appearing to work while in fact measuring inaccurately. It is vitally important that the arrow is set to zero before the measurement is made. Manual aneroid sphygmomanometers also have a permanent inaccuracy at the very highest and lowest readings. Indeed, the portable aneroid sphygmomanometer used for home visits is very inaccurate and should only be used to give 'ballpark figure' readings for assessing patients in the emergency situation, not for the treatment of hypertension. There are electronic home measurement machines available for use with a stethoscope, which are more accurate.

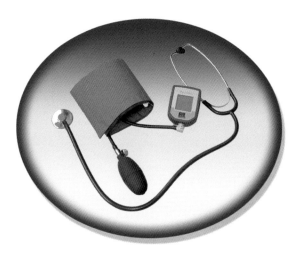

Electronic home measurement machines are available for use with a stethoscope

Automated sphygmomanometers

One concern expressed by many clinicians about automatic sphygmo-manometers is whether or not they are accurate. Some operators express disquiet that the readings can vary quite markedly when taken one after the other. If this is the case, the problem is not the machine but more likely the circumstances in which it is being used. The cuff might not be sited correctly over the brachial artery or may be the incorrect size. It might also be because the machine cannot detect Korotkoff I or V sounds due to the patient having

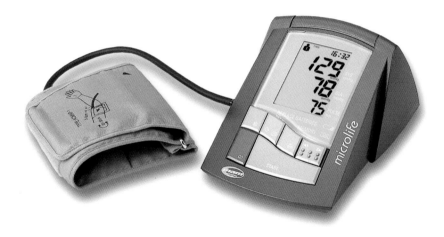

With automatic sphygmomanometers, the cuff must be sited correctly over the brachial artery and must be the correct size

an irregular pulse, as in atrial fibrillation. One other problem is if the patient is uncomfortable or tense and keeps moving. Some machines indicate if the patient moved excessively during measurement. If after re-siting the cuff, ensuring the patient is comfortable, waiting for a further 5 minutes and stressing that they should keep still, there is still a wide variation in readings, you should use an alternative instrument such as a mercury or aneroid sphygmomanometer. Some of the more expensive automatic machines offer a manual setting with which you can take the blood pressure using a stethoscope for dysrhythmic patients. Automatic devices require calibration by the supplier every 2 years.

Box 2.2

Options for measuring BP in atrial fibrillation:

• Mercury sphygmomanometer

• Manual aneroid sphygmomanometer

• Automatic sphygmomanometer with manual setting

• Electronic sphygmomanometer used with stethoscope

There are three validation standards for automatic devices: namely, the British Hypertension Society (BHS), European Society of Hypertension and the American Association for the Advancement of Medical Instrumentation (AAMI) standards. Validation of equipment is not always straightforward. The manufacturer has to approach an independent centre willing to test the device against a mercury column. That centre might take 4–5 months to test the device and then it might take up to a further year to achieve publication of a peer-reviewed paper. Only then will the BHS consider the machine for inclusion on their website. This is a slow and expensive process, which does not necessarily match the pace of technological advancement. Some manufacturers will put the machine on the market before validation is completed and others may not bother to have their machines validated at all. Nonetheless it is best to consult the BHS website (www.bhsoc.org) for up-to-date advice.

Table 2.1 BHS recommended automatic digital blood pressure devices for clinical use that are also suitable for home/self assessment, updated February 2006[2]

A&D:	767, 779 I, 787 I*, UA-774, UA-767 Plus, UA-767 PC, UA-767V, UA-767 Plus Memory, UA-767P- BT, UA-704
Microlife:	3BTO-A, 3BTO-A(2), 3AG1, As easy as 123, A100 and A100 Plus
Omron:	M5-I, 705-IT, 705-CPII, MX2 Basic, MX3 Plus, M4-I, M6-I

*International Protocol

A few automated machines are supplied with both a standard and a large cuff. If the BHS were to declare that all machines should be supplied with both cuffs, this would be a major step forward.

Wrist measurement

Many manufacturers produce wrist devices that are cheap, sold in chemist shops and intended for home measurement by the worried well. These machines are not recommended by the hypertension societies and can be inaccurate. There may, however, be a second-line place for the use of such devices in some patients including women with bilateral mastectomies and damaged lymphatics, people with nerve injury or other injuries to the upper arms, people for whom removal of any clothes is unacceptable for religious reasons and some grossly obese people for whom there is no cuff big enough. If you are using these devices it is vital that the machine is at heart level and the patient is completely still. This can be achieved either by resting the arm on pillows or by placing the thumb under the clavicle and providing support for the arm.

Box 2.3

Wrist measurement not recommended except in:

• Bilateral mastectomies

• Injury to both upper arms

• Religious/ethnic reasons

• Gross obesity

Home blood pressure measurement

Twenty-four-hour blood pressure measurement is probably the most accurate measurement you can make. It is becoming an invaluable research tool and in certain circumstances a valuable device in the assessment of some patients. As a practical, day-to-day device in general use it has severe limitations.

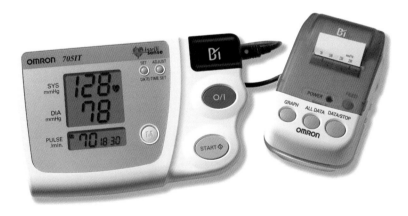

The use of a standard automatic device at home is more practical than using an ambulatory blood pressure machine

Even though prices are falling, these machines are expensive and therefore any clinic can buy only a limited number. The patient diagnosed as having white coat hypertension will need annual blood pressure measurements using the same device each time. The most efficient practice could have a turnover time only in excess of 24 hours and, hence, the realistic maximum usage in a 5-day working week is three times. Therefore one device can be used only 150 times a year.

The use of a standard automatic device by the patient at home is a more practical option. These machines are a fraction of the cost of 24-hour monitors and easy to use. My own practice has a bank of automated machines for loan to patients. The patient is instructed how to use the machine by a practice nurse or healthcare assistant and given a form inviting them to take and record eight measurements over 2 days. The form asks the patient to add all the readings, divide by eight and then add 10 mmHg to the systolic and 5 mmHg to the diastolic. This correction is vital to equate the home measurement to the 'office' measurement upon which all our science is based. (An example of the form is available in *Appendix 1*.) One alternative would be to loan a machine that includes a printer to the patient - a method already in use in some practices.

Ambulatory blood pressure monitoring

Blood pressure is a continuous haemodynamic variable. It changes in relation to stress and work rate. The hypertensive patient is someone whose resting baseline blood pressure is elevated. But when is this baseline best measured? The correct answer is 'in the middle of the night while asleep'. Some studies have suggested that identifying patients with nocturnal raised pressure correlates most accurately with subsequent morbidity.[3,4] But how do you measure this nocturnal blood pressure? The only practical method currently available is ambulatory BP monitoring. This method is, as already stated, expensive and therefore restricted to a one-off evaluation in most patients. Its true value lies in identifying the 'dipping' and 'non-dipping' patient.

We should all have a 10% reduction in baseline blood pressure at night - those that do not have this nocturnal hypotension are in the highest risk category. However, applying this test to every patient occasions a practical problem and is often confounded, with the use of present machines, by disruption to the patient's sleep. What is required is a machine that takes nocturnal readings without disturbing the patient and which is affordable in general use.

The other factor to consider is the usual surge in blood pressure in the morning, a time of day associated with an increased incidence of coronary and cerebral events. The lesson from this is to ensure that your blood pressure medication has sufficient half-life to offer 24-hour cover.

White coat hypertension

There has previously been some debate as to whether or not white coat hypertension (WCH)/isolated office hypertension exists, although it is probably becoming an accepted term. In my experience it does exist, but there is evidence to suggest that it is not a safe state of affairs and that there is excess morbidity associated with WCH in comparison with the true normotensive patient. If you do accept the diagnosis then you must treat the patient against the standard of home measurement in the same way that the patient with postural hypotension is treated against the standard of the standing blood pressure. It is valid and sensible to loan equipment or advise such patients to buy machines to use at home. It is equally important that the patients are well trained to use this equipment and know the importance of adding 10/5 mmHg to their readings.

Home measurement is accumulating a great deal of evidence in its favour. Just as self-monitoring of glucose became accepted, so too will the home measurement of blood pressure. The influential 2003 European Society of Hypertension - European Society of Cardiology (ESH-ESC) Hypertension Guidelines recommends it as a supplement to clinic readings, and a recent ESH newsletter lists its advantages succinctly.

Masked hypertension

Masked or isolated home hypertension (IHH) is a relatively new and some-what paradoxical concept. It describes the patient who has normal blood pressure in the clinic but raised blood pressure at home. This phenomenon

Table 2.2 ESH advantages of home monitoring[5]

More measurements possible

Reduces observer bias (particularly if a printer is used)

Eliminates white coat effect

Better reflection of target organ damage

Better prediction of prognosis

Improves patient compliance with treatment

Minimises placebo effect in clinical trials

has become apparent through the use of controls in studies using 24-hour ambulatory blood pressure monitoring. There is some evidence that IHH is a harmful condition and, in particular, puts the patient at increased risk of left ventricular hypertrophy. Obviously it is somewhat concealed and difficult to diagnose, but it is estimated that up to 10% of people with normal blood pressures might have this condition. Other researchers feel that with serial monitoring the figure comes down to only 1%. There is much potential here for controversy. There is also an amazing choice of names, apart from the two already quoted, such as isolated ambulatory hypertension, reverse or inverse white coat hypertension and even white coat normotension! Watch this space: we may soon be sending people with seemingly normal clinic blood pressure home with an automated blood pressure monitor, just in case!

Key points

- Automatic sphygmomanometers with brachial cuffs give the most accurate measurements as long as they are BHS recommended and used properly

- Patients with an irregular pulse require manual blood pressure measurement

- It is important to add 10/5 mmHg to home or ambulatory measurements

References

1. Medical Device Alert. MDA/2005/069, 13 December 2005

2. ww.bhsoc.org/bp_monitors/automatic.htm (accessed October 9, 2005)

3. Staessen JA, Thijs L, Fagard R et al. *JAMA* 1999;282:539-546

4. O'Brien E, Atkins A, Staessen J. *Blood Press Monit* 1996;1(suppl 1):S41-S46

5. European Society of Hypertension (ESH) Scientific Newsletter 2005;6(12r)

Chapter 3
Diagnosis and investigation

Learning objectives

This chapter will explain the initial steps taken in the newly diagnosed patient as well as follow-up investigations. You should be able to understand the basis of diagnosing the patient in terms of a primary risk factor (essential hypertension) and the separate concept of blood pressure as part of global risk stratification. The recognition of target organ damage and secondary hypertension will also be considered. The rationale and interpretation of biochemical tests and electro-cardiograms required when preparing the patient for treatment will be explained. Fundoscopy is an option for which there will be some very basic explanation.

Key words:

Appropriate investigations

Target organ damage

Secondary hypertension

Biochemistry

ECG

Fundoscopy

eGFR

Renal artery stenosis

Conn's syndrome

Phaeochromocytoma

Box 3.1

Hypertensive target organ damage:

- Left ventricular hypertrophy
- Heart failure
- Renal impairment
- Ischaemic heart disease
- Cerebrovascular disease
- Peripheral vascular disease
- Retinal changes

Box 3.2

Indications for blood pressure control:

- Moderate or severe essential hypertension (>160/100 mmHg)
- Mild essential hypertension (>140/90 mmHg) with evidence of target organ damage
- Secondary hypertension
- Diabetes or chronic kidney disease without hypertension
- Cardiovascular disease without hypertension
- Patients with high primary prevention risk scores

Diagnosis

There are various reasons why somebody might require control of their blood pressure. They may suffer from moderate primary or secondary hypertension as a standalone diagnosis, defined as a systolic pressure in excess of 160 mmHg or a diastolic pressure in excess of 100 mmHg. They may suffer from mild hypertension, a blood pressure in excess of 140 mmHg systolic or 90 mmHg diastolic, together with evidence of target organ damage such as renal impairment or hypertensive retinopathy. Pre-existing diabetes, chronic kidney disease or cardiovascular disease may dictate the need for blood pressure control without the presence of hypertension. Alternatively, they may have a high cardiovascular disease risk score, as defined by the Joint British Societies risk tables, or even evidence of metabolic syndrome *(risk assessment is explained in Chapter 7)*.

The assessment of the patient requires a systematic approach involving a series of blood pressure measurements over a set period of time, as well as a history, physical examination, blood tests and ECG. The most sensible approach to this is to have a written protocol in the practice based on established guidelines such as those offered by the British Hypertension Society or Joint British Societies. A practice-based protocol will conform to locally available resources and gives a sense of ownership. It ensures that all those working in this field 'sing from the same hymn sheet' and that for each patient all the necessary steps are taken regardless of who carries out the assessment. Usually it is the nurses who particularly like to have a protocol upon which they can act and invariably they are the ones who actually follow them correctly. The Whitby Group Practice Hypertension Protocol is available in *Appendix 2* as one example of how this might be done and a more detailed discussion of protocols is given in *Chapter 8*. It is very important that such protocols are updated on a regular basis. Measurement of blood pressure was described in *Chapter 2*.

History and examination

The most important part of the history involves basic questions about smoking and alcohol consumption, as the former confers additional risk of cardiovascular disease and the latter will have a direct effect on blood pressure itself. Smoking history should include not just whether or not a person smokes but also how many units and for how long. If the patient is now a non-smoker, past consumption should be estimated. The best means of describing a smoker is in terms of 'pack years' where the number of cigarettes is equated to packs of 20 and if they smoke 40 per day the total years of smoking is doubled. The person who recently stopped smoking cannot be considered a non-smoker in terms of insurance evaluations until 1 year after cessation and in terms of risk assessment it is 5 years after stopping.

Excess alcohol consumption is not always easy to evaluate. People are often reticent to admit to their true consumption and can often underestimate that consumption quite markedly. The effects of alcohol on cardiovascular risk are uncertain, but what is clear is that heavy consumption, especially binge drinking, will increase the patient's blood pressure in the 48 hours following the drinking session.

Certain prescription medications such as the contraceptive pill and both steroidal and non-steroidal anti-inflammatories will increase blood pressure.

A family history of cardiovascular disease in a first-degree male relative aged less than 55 years or female relative aged less than 65 increases primary cardiovascular risk by a factor of 1.5.

With examination, as with history, it is the simple factors that are most important, in particular the patients' weight, height and abdominal circumference. The pulse rate and rhythm are vital at every assessment, and one drawback of using automated sphygmomanometers is that we often forget to feel the pulse and might therefore miss an irregular rhythm.

At initial assessment of the heart sounds makes sense as you might rarely pick up a murmur, particularly an aortic systolic murmur. It is also useful to check the foot pulses in somebody at risk of peripheral arterial disease, as this may give a clue to the presence of renal artery stenosis. More detailed examination is likely to be helpful only in very specific cases.

Fundoscopy

As hypertension is better diagnosed and treated these days, hypertensive retinopathy is becoming less common. It is more likely that an optician rather than a general practitioner will pick up any changes.

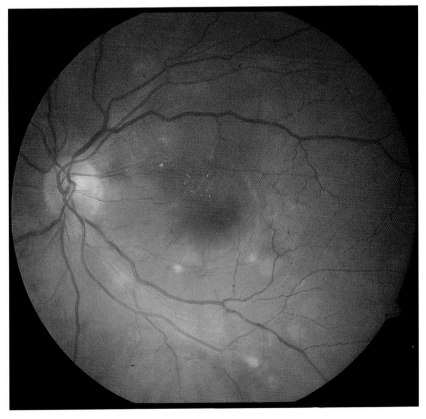

Figure 3.1 'Fundoscopy - don't bother'
This photograph shows a grade 2 to 3 hypertensive retinopathy with AV crossing signs, cotton wool spots, flame shaped haemorrhages in the nerve fibre layer and macula exudation but no disc oedema

Reproduced with the kind permission of Mr J van der Hoek of Scarborough Hospital

There is no place for routine fundoscopy in the hypertensive patient in primary care. Few practitioners have the necessary skills to perform accurate fundoscopy and, even if they did, the lack of regular pathological findings in hypertensive patients would blunt them in time. A recent review of

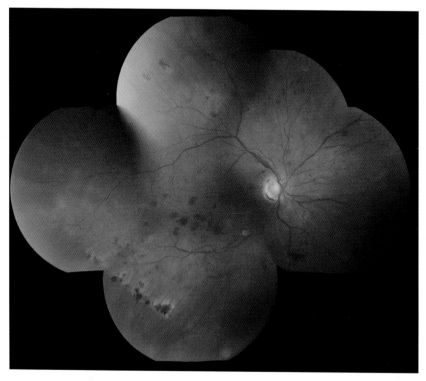

Figure 3.2 'Fundoscopy - malignant hypertension is now very rare'
This photograph shows a grade 2 to 3 diabetic retinopathy showing AV signs,
dot blot haemorrhages, venous bleeding and pre-retinal haemorrhage in a
patient with malignant hypertension

Reproduced with the kind permission of Mr J van der Hoek of Scarborough Hospital

111 reports came to the conclusion that there was wide observer variability
in fundoscopy, poor predictive value in such examinations and overlap of
pathology with other disease states. The report concluded that there was
little additional value in routine fundoscopy of hypertensive patients.[1] It
found consistent value only in fundoscopy of patients who had suffered a
stroke. It advised that we look for cotton wool spots, hard exudates and flame

haemorrhage only, not microvascular changes. In other words, act on grade III changes and ignore grade I and II - so forget arterial narrowing completely.

If despite this you want to look at the fundi it is really best performed by dilatating the pupil, especially in the elderly. Imagine that you are looking at a wall of vessels and systematically work your way out from the optic disc in each quartile of the fundi. Malignant hypertension is now very rare, thanks to improvements in the diagnosis and treatment of hypertension; you are therefore very unlikely to detect papilloedema.

Blood investigations

Box 3.3

Initial blood investigations - all patients:

- FBC
- U&Es
- Random blood glucose
- LFTs
  - gamma GT
  - uric acid
- Non-fasting total and HDL cholesterols

At initial assessment *(see box 3.3)* a full blood count is useful because it makes sense to screen for blood dyscrasia in cardiovascular disease. Urea, creatinine and electrolytes are an absolute must to screen for renal disease. They are also vital prior to the use of diuretics, angiotensin-converting enzyme (ACE) inhibitors or angiotensin receptor blockers (ARBs), as well as important in the subsequent follow-up of patients using these drugs. The gamma GT will pick up the occasional well-hidden alcohol problem and LFTs may be needed prior to prescription of a statin. Gout is a relative contraindication to the use of thiazide diuretics. Total cholesterol and HDL-cholesterol are needed as part of the overall cardiovascular risk assessment.

In terms of follow-up, glucose should be performed annually and urea, creatinine and electrolytes are necessary only if the patient is taking a diuretic, ACE inhibitor or ARB.

Urine investigations

Urinalysis for protein is useful at both assessment and follow-up because renal disease is a cause of hypertension as well as a consequence of it. Glycosuria is a late finding in diabetes and in this day and age is unacceptable as a screening test. Instead random blood glucose should be performed annually in all patients receiving treatment for raised blood pressure, and a raised result should lead to further investigation with either two fasting blood glucoses or a glucose tolerance test.

Electrocardiography

Electrocardiography should be available to all UK general practices. Many practices have interpretive machines while some rely on a hospital-based service. Interpretive machines are on the whole very reliable. They are set-up to over-report abnormalities as a safety feature. Therefore a 'normal' report is usually accurate, but abnormal reports are sometimes unjustified. It is important that human eyes verify the report. Many GPs feel they are insufficiently trained and experienced to do this, which is an unfortunate attitude to take. If you routinely look at every ECG generated for your patients and follow some basic rules, you will soon become experienced. Nobody will expect you to have the skills of a cardiologist; we are all judged by our likely level of competence (or incompetence) compared with our peers.

The basic rules are that you always look at the rate first, rhythm second and the existence of P waves and PR interval third. By doing this you have done more than half the job already. You will have excluded bradycardia, tachycardia, heart block and any arrhythmia. Now look at the individual complexes for signs of obvious ischaemia or, more importantly in terms of hypertension, left ventricular hypertrophy (LVH). Evidence of old ischaemia might be detected by the existence of Q waves in leads III and aVf. Abnormal ST or T wave changes in the ventricular leads will suggest current ischaemia. The more ECGs you look at, the better you will get at spotting the changes: it comes down to self-discipline in the main.

LVH is often a relatively easy diagnosis to make. It can be defined on an ECG as where the sum of the highest ventricular R wave in V5 or V6 and lowest ventricular S wave in V1 or V2 comes to a total that is greater than 35 mm and there is T wave inversion in V5 and V6. By changing the 35 mm to a higher figure such as 37 mm you can make your ECG diagnosis more specific and less sensitive, as I have done in our practice protocol (see *Appendix 2*). Patients with ECG evidence of hypertrophy deserve a follow-up echocardiogram to confirm the diagnosis. LVH is highly predictive of future events when applied to global risk assessment *(see Chapter 7).*

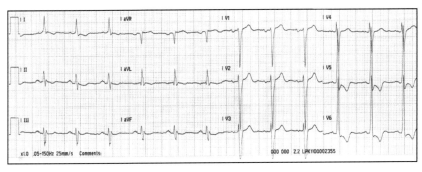

Figure 3.3 ECG of left ventricular hypertrophy

Reproduced with the kind permission of Dr Phil Batin, Pinderfields and Pontefract NHS Trust

Special investigations for secondary causes of hypertension

The two common secondary causes of hypertension are renal failure and primary aldosteronism/Conn's syndrome. The former is easier to diagnose and more difficult to treat than the latter.

Box 3.4

eGFR = estimated glomerular filtration rate:

• GFR is the percentage of remaining renal function

• The laboratory estimates eGFR using age, gender, serum creatinine and +/- black race

• Black people have a higher muscle bulk therefore higher serum creatinine than white and Asian people, thus we multiply eGFR by 1.2

• Laboratory requests must detail race, sex and age

Box 3.5

The National Service Framework for Renal Services, Part Two: Chronic kidney disease, acute renal failure and end of life care:

'4.7 The area where this Quality Requirement (QR) is likely to bring about the greatest change is in the choice of test of kidney function. This QR aims to improve the accuracy of testing, and hence reduce the number of people with undiagnosed Chronic Kidney Disease (CKD), by changing the standard measure of the kidney's filtration function from serum creatinine (SCr) alone to estimated glomerular filtration rate (eGFR)'

'4.8 Improved detection of CKD using eGFR will mean that more people have their CKD detected at an early stage. A Canadian study (Duncan et al) found that of 2,781 outpatients referred by community physicians to an urban laboratory network for SCr measurement, 182 (0.65%) had both abnormal SCr and abnormal eGFR ($\leq$50 ml/min), but a further 387 patients (14%) had normal SCr and abnormal eGFR. These findings suggest that simply switching from SCr to eGFR could cause the number of cases of stage 3 and 4 CKD detected to approximately triple, even without any increase in the numbers of people tested'

Renal disease is diagnosed by evidence of protein in the urine, raised serum creatinine or low estimated glomerular filtration rate (eGFR) (*see box 3.4*). Creatinine clearance is a complicated test seldom used in general practice.

eGFR is the gold standard, as recommended in the National Service Framework for Renal Services (*see box 3.5*). In this latest NSF, the term 'Chronic Kidney Disease' (CKD) is used rather than 'Chronic Renal Failure' (CRF). The use of eGFR will triple the detection of CKD, allowing earlier, and therefore more effective, treatment of this disorder. The introduction of eGFR was highlighted by its inclusion in the 2006 Quality Outcomes Framework Indicators for CKD.

While kidney failure will become easier to spot, renal artery stenosis (RAS) will remain difficult. Suspicion of this condition should be raised by the existence of peripheral atherosclerosis and especially intermittent claudication. Examination of the leg pulses and particularly leg dopplers may be useful. Existence of a femoral and especially a renal bruit are strongly suspicious, but these are examinations a primary care physician is not going to perform routinely nor with much confidence. RAS is usually picked up following a rapid rise in creatinine after initiation of low dose ACE inhibitors. Abdominal ultrasound may show unilateral or bilateral small kidneys or even an associated abdominal aortic aneurysm. RAS can be best diagnosed by renal arteriogram but this test is unavailable to secondary care as well as primary care in many centres.

Box 3.6

Suspect renal artery stenosis (RAS) in patients with:

- Peripheral atherosclerosis
- Femoral or renal bruit
- Rise in creatinine with ACE inhibitors
- Small kidneys on ultrasound scan

Primary aldosteronism is undoubtedly quite common and seldom diagnosed. **Conn's syndrome** describes aldosteronism secondary to an adrenal tumour but is often mistakenly used to refer to primary aldosteronism. It can be very difficult to obtain an accurate diagnosis. Finding low serum potassium in a patient with severe hypertension that is resistant to treatment raises suspicion. Spiral computerised axial tomograpy (CAT) scan may detect an adrenal tumour but the aldosterone-secreting tissue may be remote from the adrenal gland and may be found in numerous other sites of glandular tissue. The detection of an abnormal serum renin:aldosterone ratio makes for a definitive diagnosis. It is no longer necessary to take the patient off all antihypertensive medication to investigate this condition, as was the case previously. Then it was a potentially dangerous procedure that had to be performed as a hospital inpatient investigation. It required a lengthy admission and even then no definitive answer was necessarily found (*see Chapter 11*).

A more pragmatic, less scientific, less purist, but potentially safer alternative is to assume the diagnosis might be primary aldosteronism or Conn's syndrome and simply try an aldosterone antagonist such as spironolactone. If the blood pressure is controlled, then just perform a CAT scan and leave it at that. Note that spironolactone does not have a license for hypertension treatment in the UK but is licensed for the treatment of primary aldosteronism. As a generic drug with no major pharmaceutical company willing to fund research or a new license application this situation is unlikely to change. You must inform the patient you are using the drug 'off-licence'.

Finally we should consider **phaeochromocytomas**, medullary adrenal gland tumours that secrete the catecholamines adrenaline and noradrenaline (epinephrine and norepinephrine). Ten percent of phaeochromocytomas are extra-medullary. Anyone working in one of the specialist centres might be forgiven for thinking such tumours are common, but most primary care practices will never see a case despite often looking for them. Clinically they are suspected in young patients who have severe, sometimes labile, hypertension that is resistant to treatment. Such patients often have associated tachycardia, palpitations, headaches and, classically, anxiety attacks. The diagnosis of this condition is usually made by collecting a 24-hour urine specimen for vanillylmandelic acid (VMA), although some centres use serum catecholamine tests. Twenty-five percent of cases are currently diagnosed by chance during routine abdominal CT scanning for unrelated indications.[2] Pre-surgery treatment is with alpha-blockers initially and then beta-blockers later. Phenoxybenzamine is a non-competitive alpha adrenoceptor-blocker, and this confers an advantage over the other agents in the class. Beta-blockers such as propranolol or atenolol should be added later, as unopposed alpha-receptor stimulation can cause a hypertensive crisis. For this reason labetalol, a combined alpha- and beta-blocker with greater beta activity, is no longer the initial drug of choice. Dihydropyridine calcium channel blockers are the ideal third-line treatment.

Key points

- Routine fundoscopy is unhelpful and unnecessary

- Left ventricular hypertrophy is easy to diagnose on ECG

- Estimated glomerular filtration rate (eGFR) is the gold standard for early detection of renal failure

- Primary aldosteronism is common and can either be an assumed diagnosis or confirmed by measuring the serum renin:aldosterone ratio

References

1. Van den Born B, Hulsman C, Hoekstra J. *BMJ* 2005;331:73-76

2. Lenders J, Eisenhofer G, Mannelli M. *Lancet* 2005;366(9486):665-675

Chapter 4

Lifestyle advice

Learning objectives

We all recognise the importance of lifestyle in terms of health, but we usually feel it is an uphill task imposing restrictions on patients. It does not need to be like that. This chapter introduces you to the principles of organising effective lifestyle advice that is pragmatic and sensible. The cycle of change will be explained. The use of advice sheets and personalised planning will be outlined. Above all you should feel ready to prepare your own specific strategy for your patients. Remember that non-pharmacological interventions alone are recommended for the patient with mild hypertension.

Key words:

Motivation

Cycle of change

Healthy eating

Salt avoidance

Smoking cessation

Exercise

Motivation

Never underestimate the influence of the word of a doctor or nurse. Many people will stop smoking or lose weight simply because they were given sincere advice by a healthcare worker. Equally there is a risk that failure to achieve the advised goals can lead to the patient becoming demoralised and feeling unworthy because they let the doctor down. This in turn can make them reluctant to attend appointments and can affect adherence to medication. We all have to be careful not to make the patient feel guilty.

Dire warnings of impending doom if lifestyle advice is not adhered to are unnecessary for most patients and probably counterproductive. Most people in society are aware of the consequences of a poor lifestyle but feel they cannot achieve change. Convincing them that they can change is the key to success. Realistic goals are required as well as simple methods. Making the patient part of the planning process avoids the feeling that you are making them do something that they do not want to do themselves. Enlisting the help of friends and family is often useful. If you have patients who have successfully stopped smoking or lost weight consider asking them to champion the cause.

Using locally developed advice leaflets gives a sense of ownership. Patients will respect literature with your name, or the practice name, on it more than something that is seen as nationally based. In this age of computerisation it is easy to set up a folder of Microsoft Word documents providing simple advice in just one or two A4 sheets with your name at the end. Alternatively, use the system based on your practice computer - for example, the Mentor System on EMIS. The advice leaflets on Mentor can be copied and pasted into Word documents and then personalised or, for the ultimate in computer patient-personalised sophistication, you could combine them in a mail merge document. If you do this it is important to also copy the Mentor copyright and acknowledge it as your source. Examples of how I have adapted Mentor advice leaflets are included at the end of this chapter *(box 4.4 and table 4.4)*

Motivation has to be repetitive. Lifestyle encouragement has to be systematically repeated and is an integral part of the biannual follow up.

Cycle of change[1]

The cycle has six steps.

Recognition is the realisation that something has to change. This might occur because of a personal decision, advice from a health professional or the discovery of disease in the individual or even another member of the family.

Information is the step where further clarification is sought or provided. This might be through a patient information leaflet, the Internet or a television broadcast.

Planning is the preparation of a plan of action to deal with the situation and ideally is personalised.

Action is the point at which change takes place.

Change describes the period after action when the outcome might be successful or a failure. The change might be perceived as beneficial or counterproductive by the individual and this is a key stage where total failure may occur. Support is vital.

Contentment is the final result of the action. The individual might be contentedly successful or even contentedly a failure.

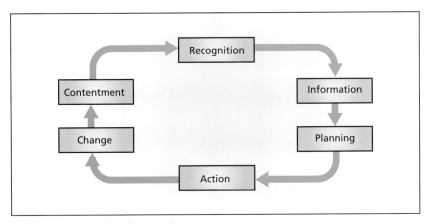

Figure 4.1 The cycle of change[1]

The primary care team might become involved at any stage. We may be pointing out the need for change or the patient might approach us for advice having initially decided to do something or they may have failed in their own attempt to change. The process is a cycle, not a circle; it is not closed at 'contentment' and the recognition that change was needed has to be continually reinforced.

Diet

Box 4.1

Ten top tips on successful dieting:

1. Have a practice plan/protocol that includes timelines

2. 10% or 10 kg is a reasonable target: be realistic

3. Three meals a day and no snacks is the most important advice

4. Use small plates and do not refill them

5. The patient that asks for help is most likely to succeed and deserves all the help you can provide

6. Use scales that go up to 200 kg or 30 stones

7. Use a successful patient as a champion

8. Join forces with local slimming clubs and gyms

9. Have a customised healthy eating sheet, not a diet sheet

10. Before prescribing weight reduction drugs get the patient to lose some weight to show willing

---

Weight reduction will reduce blood pressure directly but, more importantly, will lessen overall cardiovascular disease risk.

Table 4.1 Body Mass Index (BMI) kg/m² and Waist Circumference (WC)		
BMI		
	Caucasian	Asian
Normal	<25	<23
Overweight	25 to <30	23 to <28
Obese	30 to <35	28 to <33
Grossly obese	≥35	≥33
WC		
Men	<102 cms	<92 cms
Women	<88 cms	<78 cms

A weight loss of 10 kg or 10% of current weight (whichever is greater) is a realistic achievement for most people and will reduce their systolic blood pressure by 10 mmHg. This will make them feel better about themselves and is sufficient to improve their health. Over-ambitious targets should be avoided. If the patient is very keen to lose more weight they should take the 'one step at a time' approach. It is important to record the current and target weights and write them down for the patient (*see box 4.4*). You might wish to include a patient-held record of weight loss. Emphasise the point that successful diets work slowly and reflect a culture change in eating. Crash diets are pointless. The idea is to get the weight down and keep it down.

The most important single tip is that we should all eat three times a day - no more, no less and no snacking. It is not just how much we eat, but also the quality of the food we eat that counts. The patient should be encouraged to eat at least five portions of fruit or vegetable daily (but in essence as much as they like). A portion should be the size of their clenched fist. The best time to eat fruit is at the start of the meal, so that they fill themselves up. I advise patients that they should use a low fat diet. They should also be encouraged to eat oily fish on two occasions a week.

Shopping is a key factor in dieting. It is often best to advise the shopper or cook more than the patient. Healthy shopping is more about looking at the labels and avoiding foods high in unsaturated fats rather than counting calories. Because we are human it is okay to cheat as long as it is done in a disciplined fashion. Cheating must be restricted to one treat a week. This approach really works. The Harvard DASH (Dietary Approaches to Stop Hypertension) diet allows as much fruits and vegetables as the patient likes, along with a low salt and fat intake.[2] It is specifically designed to help people lose weight and lower blood pressure and is similar to the diet described in these pages.

Patients who are obese or grossly obese need a little more help. This might be in the form of drugs such as orlistat or sibutramine. Treatment with sibu-tramine is not recommended for individuals whose blood pressure before start of therapy is above 145/90 mmHg. Treatment should be discontinued in people whose blood pressure rises above 145/90 mmHg. It is contraindi-cated in uncontrolled hypertension. It is vitally important to follow the NICE Guidelines (22 for orlistat [table 4.2] and 31 for sibutramine) when using these drugs; failure to do so not only wastes money but also the patient's time. In particular it is important to insist that patients lose some weight before they start on the drug - only that way can you ensure that they are modifying their diet.

If all else fails, the grossly obese patient should be considered for barometric surgery. The technique of placing adjustable bands around the stomach via the laparoscope is safe and effective when performed by skilled surgeons and anaesthetists. These patients often have very low life quality as well as poor longevity and such surgery could be seen as life saving.

Table 4.2 NICE Technology Appraisal Guidance 22:
Orlistat for the treatment of obesity in adults

Orlistat should be prescribed for people who have lost at least 2.5 kg in weight by diet and physical activity alone in the month prior to the first prescription

Patients should have a BMI $\geq$28 kg/m^2 plus comorbidities - eg type 2 diabetes, high blood pressure and/or high total cholesterol level BMI of 30 kg/m^2 or more with no associated comorbidities

When treatment with orlistat is offered, arrangements should be made for appropriate health professionals to offer specific advice, support and counselling on diet, physical activity and behavioural strategies

Orlistat should be prescribed only for people between the ages of 18 and 75 years

Continuation of therapy beyond 3 months should be supported by evidence of a loss of at least a further 5% of body weight from the start of drug treatment

Continuation of therapy beyond 6 months should be supported by evidence of a cumulative weight loss of at least 10% of body weight from the start of drug treatment

Treatment should not usually be continued beyond 12 months, and never beyond 24 months

There is no evidence to support the co-prescribing of orlistat and sibutramine

Salt

Salt is specifically implicated in hypertension and the patient should be advised to significantly reduce salt intake by avoiding foods with high salt content and never adding salt to food. Salt substitutes such as 'low salt' can be used as long as it is in moderation. Processed foods are responsible for about 75% of the salt we consume and therefore reading labels carefully is helpful.

Many antacids contain salt and therefore care is required in their use. The *British National Formulary* indicates which antacids have high salt content.

Box 4.2

Foods high in salt:

- Anchovies
- Bacon
- Baked beans
- Biscuits
- Bread
- Breakfast cereals
- Cheese
- Chips
- Cooking sauces
- Gravy granules
- Hot chocolate
- Olives
- Pickles

- Pizza
- Pretzels
- Ready meals
- Salted fish
- Salted nuts
- Sausages
- Smoked foods
- Soup
- Soy sauce
- Stock cubes
- Tinned spaghetti
- Tinned vegetables/pulses
- Yeast extract

Food Standards Agency Website: www.food.gov.uk/aboutus/fsawebsites/

The Second Joint British Society Guidelines (JBS 2) recommend a daily limit of less than 100 mmol/l of salt (*table 4.3*).[3] Adherence to this limit will bring about a small reduction in blood pressure.

Table 4.3 Second Joint British Society Guidelines lifestyle recommendations[2]

Stop smoking completely

Total intake of fat ≤30% of total energy intake

Intake of saturated fats to ≤30% of total fat intake

Intake of dietary cholesterol <300 mg/day

Replace saturated fats by an increased intake of monounsaturated fats

Increase intake of fresh fruit and vegetables to at least 5 portions per day

Regular intake of fish and other sources of omega 3 fatty acids (at least 2 servings of fish per week)

Limit alcohol intake to <21 units per week (men) and <14 units per week (women)

Limit intake of salt to <100 mmol/l per day (<6 g of sodium chloride or <2.4 g of sodium per day)

Regular aerobic physical activity of at least 30 minutes per day, most days of the week, should be taken (eg fast walking/swimming)

Alcohol

There is great debate about whether alcohol is beneficial or harmful in cardiovascular disease but that debate is around mild-to-moderate consumption. Obviously heavy consumption is quite simply bad for you. Binge drinking has a temporary hypertensive effect. Most people do not recognise their level of alcohol consumption. Consider asking the patient to keep an alcohol diary for a week, recording a small glass of wine as one unit and a pint of ordinary beer as two units of alcohol. This may well be an eye-opener for them.

Smoking

Smoking adds to the overall risk of cardiovascular disease and it is important to keep reminding patients that they must stop. The new General Medical Services Contract requires that we ask hypertension patients about their smoking habits at least once every 15 months if they are a smoker or ex-smoker. Those who have never smoked do not need to be asked more than once. Those who smoke must be encouraged to stop and offered help to stop. Help can be by way of a smoking cessation clinic and might include the prescription of nicotine replacement therapy or bupropion.

For some, particularly women, you might try to appeal to their altruistic side by mentioning the effects of passive smoking.

Box 4.3

Tips on stopping smoking:

- Set a memorable date to stop

- Calculate how much money will be saved

- Chewing gum or carrots

- Ask friends not to offer cigarettes

- Consider the effect of passive smoking on other people

- Use nicotine replacement therapy

- Join a smoking cessation clinic

Stopping smoking is most successful if the patient has a genuine desire to stop. They should be encouraged to attend a clinic rather than just take medication. If they fail they should be encouraged to try again. Tips for stopping might include setting a date that is easy to remember such as the first of the month or an anniversary so that they can easily recall how long they have stopped for. Calculation of how much money will be saved is a powerful motivation. If they want something to do with their mouth try chewing gum or carrots. They should prepare themselves to resist at times of weakness, especially if alcohol is involved, by asking their friends to not offer them cigarettes.

Point out to them that it is never too late to stop and that the risks associated with smoking diminish quite rapidly after cessation.

Exercise

Modern life not only offers fast food, salt and cigarettes but also is too easy. Cars, washing machines and television sets have made us sedentary. The other side of the coin is that we are 'too busy' to find time to exercise. The patient must be repeatedly encouraged to find time to exercise for 30 minutes on at least five occasions per week. Point out that exercise increases the amount of 'good' cholesterol (HDL-C). The exercise should ideally be sustained but equally an accumulation of 30 minutes is of value and so advice like 'use the stairs at work' is useful. An example of good exercise is a continuous brisk walk, but what form the exercise takes does not really matter; it mainly needs to be something the patient enjoys. For younger patients the exercise should be more demanding - for example, jogging or cycling.

Fears that vigorous exercise is dangerous should be dismissed. Regular aerobic exercise reduces the risk of cardiovascular disease; cardiovascular events suffered during exercise were probably going to occur at rest anyway.

Having said all of the above, there is a place for rest as well. The patient who has type A personality and never stops is also at risk. Therefore for some individuals it can be prudent to advise them to put aside time for relaxation as well as exercise.

Box 4.4

Changing your diet and losing weight in a sensible, healthy way:

Your weight is .... kg .... stones

Minus 10 kg or 10% equals your target weight of .... kg .... stones

Think of it in terms of changing over to a healthy way of eating when you will enjoy food in a different way. You are more likely to stay slimmer if you keep to the habits learned. As soon as you start to lose weight you will start to feel better about yourself

- Eat three meals a day and don't skip meals. This will just make you feel more hungry and think about food more. You will be more likely to overeat in the evening

- Use small plates and don't refill them. Don't eat seconds

- Don't pick at food and snacks during the day. You won't feel the satisfaction of a good meal and it's amazing how these calories mount up and are forgotten about. In the same way don't eat leftovers

- Enjoy your food! If you eat small regular meals without picking between them you should have a healthy appetite. Healthy food can be just as enjoyable as fattening food and after a while you may find your tastes changing

- Keep your alcohol intake to a minimum, as most alcoholic drinks contain lots of calories

- Drink plenty of fluids but watch your intake of milk in tea and coffee. Have no more than half a pint of skimmed or semi-skimmed milk a day. Other drinks should be sugar free

- Increase the amount of exercise you do. Excess weight will come off more quickly and will be more likely to stay off the more you do. You will also feel fitter and less tired. You should have 30 minutes of continuous, vigorous exercise on 5 days of every week

- The aim of your diet is to increase the amount of fibre and starchy foods and reduce the amount of saturated fat and refined sugars you eat

- Try to eat vegetables or fruit at every meal. They provide valuable vitamins, minerals and fibre with little fat. Try to aim for five portions of fruit or vegetables a day

- Your fat intake should be kept to a minimum using the following tips. Use low fat spreads sparingly. Measure out oil. Grill instead of fry where possible. Cut excess fat off meat and choose the leaner cuts in smaller portions. Avoid the fatty meats, sausages and mince. Use low calorie dressings and low fat mayonnaise on salads

- Cheese, milk and yoghurt contain lots of calcium. Try to switch to the lower fat versions, which have the same calcium content but fewer calories

- You should only cheat for one meal a week

Extract copyright EMIS. New diets available from www.webmentorlibrary.com

Table 4.4 Low fat healthy eating sheet

Foods that can be eaten regularly (little or no fat and/or 'healthy' foods)

Cereal foods Wholemeal flour and bread. Porridge oats. High fibre breafast cereals. Wholegrain rice and pasta

Fruit, veg and nuts All fresh and frozen vegetables and fruit. Dried beans and lentils. Baked potatoes. Dried fruit. Walnuts

Fish All white fish. Oily fish such as herrings, mackerel, sardines, kippers, pilchards, or salmon (not tinned in oil)

Meat Lean white meat, such as chicken and turkey breast (without skin)

Eggs, dairy foods Skimmed or semi-skimmed milk. Cottage or curd cheese. Low fat yoghurt. Egg whites

Fats and spreads None

Drinks and soups Tea and coffee. Mineral water. Fruit juices

Foods to be eaten in moderation

Cereal foods White flour and bread. Low fibre breakfast cereals. White rice and pasta. Plain biscuits. Plain or fruit scones

Fruit, veg and nuts Oven chips. Avocado pears. Olives. Almonds. Pecans. Hazelnuts

Fish Shellfish

Meat Lean ham, beef, pork, and lamb. Lean mince. Liver and kidney

Eggs, dairy foods Edam. Camembert. Parmesan. Up to 3 egg yolks a week

Fats and spreads Low fat spreads. Margarine (high in polyunsaturates). Corn, sunflower and olive oil

Drinks and soups Packet soups. Alcoholic drinks

Table 4.4 Low fat healthy eating sheet (continued)

Foods to avoid or to eat rarely (high in fat and/or 'unhealthy' foods)

Cereal foods Croissants. Fried bread. Most cakes and biscuits. Pastries. Suet pudding

Fruit, veg and nuts Chips. Fried or roast potatoes. Fried, creamed, buttered or cheesed vegetables. Crisps and potato snacks. Coconut. Brazils. Roasted peanuts

Fish Fish roe. Caviar

Meat Visible fat on meat. Crackling. Sausages. Patés. Duck, goose. Meat pies/pasties

Eggs, dairy foods Whole milk. Cream. Ice cream. Most hard cheeses. Chocolate. Cream cheese

Fats and spreads Butter. Dripping and lard. Margarine not high in polyunsaturates

Drinks and soups Cream soups. Milky drinks. Sugary drinks

Extract copyright EMIS and PiP 2006, as distributed on www.patient.co.uk and www.webmentorlibrary.com

Key points

- Repetitive motivation from healthcare professionals is effective in promoting a healthy lifestyle

- Mild hypertension (140/90-159/99 mmHg) requires lifestyle advice

- A weight loss of 10 kg will reduce systolic blood pressure by 10 mmHg

References

1. Prochaska JO, DiClemente CC, Norcross JC. In search of how people change. *Am Psychol* 1992;47:1102-1104.

2. Moore TJ, Vollmer WM, Appel LJ et al. *Hypertension* 1999;34(3):472-477

3. Joint British Societies. *Heart* 2005;91:(suppl V):v1-v52

Chapter 5

Therapeutics

Learning objectives

This chapter will discuss the different groups of therapeutic agents used to treat hypertension. We will cover how they work, when to use them and when not to use them. Side effects are an important aspect of drug therapy and particularly relevant to compliance. Polypharmacy is commonly required and therefore the interaction of these drugs with each other and other agents is covered.

Key words:

ABCD Guidelines

Bradykinase

Synergism

Atenolol controversy

Dihydropyridine

Fixed-dose reaction

Aldosteronism

Centrally acting antihypertensive

ABCD

The fourth British Hypertension Society Guidelines (BHS IV) suggest the use of the ABCD system.[1] I use this system in my own prescribing practice and feel it works extremely well because it leads the prescriber to use synergistic combinations in a logical manner. We shall examine the drugs used to treat hypertension by following the same commonsense pathway.

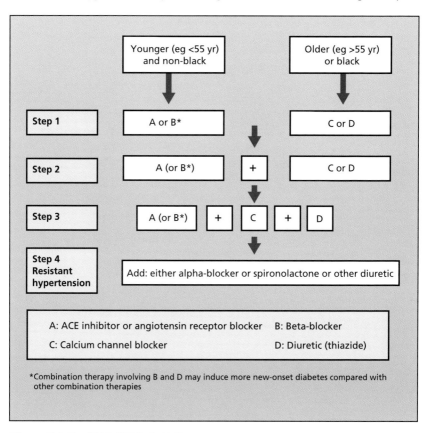

Figure 5.1 The BHS ABCD Guidelines

Reproduced, with the kind permission of the Journal of Human Hypertension and the British Hypertension Society, from Brown MJ, British Hypertension Society. J Human Hypertens 2003;17:81-86

A is for angiotensin-converting enzyme inhibitors or angiotensin receptor blockers

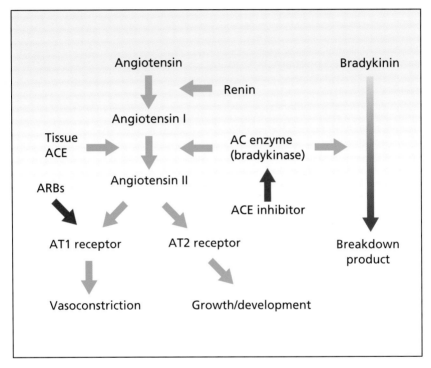

Figure 5.2 The renin-angiotensin system and the breakdown of bradykinin

Angiotensin-converting enzyme (ACE) inhibitors were first used in the early 1980s for the treatment of both hypertension and heart failure. Angiotensin receptor blockers (ARBs) became available about 10 years later. They both act on the renin-angiotensin system. ACE inhibitors block the angiotensin-converting enzyme, thereby reducing the production of angiotensin II. This restricts the vasoconstriction caused by stimulation of the AT1 receptor. The angiotensin system influences growth - hence the contraindication of these drugs in pregnancy. The angiotensin-converting enzyme is also called bradykinase as it promotes the breakdown of bradykinin. This is both a help and a hindrance as the bradykinin build-up reduces blood pressure due to its vasodilatory properties but also causes a dry cough because most of this activity is in pulmonary tissue.

Box 5.1

ACE inhibitor hypertension doses:

- Captopril: 25 mg bd to 50 mg tds
- Cilazapril: 0.5 mg to 5 mg od
- Enalapril: 2.5 mg to 20 mg od or bd
- Fosinopril: 10 mg to 20 mg od or bd
- Imidapril: 2.5 mg to 20 mg od
- Lisinopril: 2.5 mg to 20 mg od or bd
- Moexipril: 3.75 mg to 15 mg od or bd
- Perindopril: 2 mg to 8 mg od
- Quinapril: 2.5 mg to 40 mg od or bd
- Ramipril: 1.25 mg to 10 mg od
- Trandolapril: 0.5 mg to 2 mg od or bd

The ARBs have a more selective action in that they directly block the AT1 receptor. Therefore they do not cause a bradykinin build-up and no ACE inhibitor cough. In fact their selective action means they have very few side effects and this sets them apart from most hypertension treatments. They are therefore very useful in the patient who is non-compliant with treatment. This lack of bradykinin vasodilatation is made up for by the fact that ARBs block the angiotensin II stimulation completely, even that caused by tissue angiotensin-converting enzyme. When you change a patient onto an ARB because of an 'ACE inhibitor cough' it is important to warn them that it can take up to 8 weeks for the cough to settle.

Box 5.2

ARB hypertension doses:

- Candesartan: 2 mg to 32 mg od
- Eprosartan: 300 mg to 400 mg od or bd
- Irbesartan: 75 mg to 300 mg od
- Losartan: 25 mg to 100 mg od
- Olmesartan: 10 mg to 40 mg od
- Telmisartan: 40 mg to 80 mg od
- Valsartan: 40 mg to 160 mg od

The patient in whom hypertension is caused by the renin factor is more likely to be younger. Afro-Caribbean patients are less likely to be hypertensive due to this renin factor. Hence the ABCD table recommendation that initiation of treatment with ACE inhibitors and ARBs should be in the non-black patient aged under 55 years.

Both these classes of drugs are particularly useful in patients who have left ventricular failure following myocardial infarction, left ventricular hypertrophy, diabetes and diabetic nephropathy. They are both also useful in migraine sufferers. The ARBs have been shown to reduce the onset of diabetes.

ARBs and ACE inhibitors are contraindicated in pregnancy, aortic stenosis and renal artery stenosis. Hypersensitivity reactions to ACE inhibitors are rare but can be dangerous if they involve marked facial and oral angioedema. They usually develop slowly over 1-2 weeks and therefore the association with the drug may not be immediately obvious. A recent controversial meta-analysis has suggested that the renal protection of ACE inhibitors or ARBs is due more to the antihypertensive effect rather than any direct influence,[2] and no doubt the subject will be revisited many times long after this book is published.

Initiation of therapy can result in postural hypotension, but this is rarely the case in hypertension and more of a problem in the hypotensive heart failure patient. I usually advise patients to take the first dose on retiring to bed because of the risk of their blood pressure falling rapidly and making them 'feel dizzy'. Alternatively you can ask them to take the first tablet with plenty of water while sitting down and to remain sitting for 2 hours. It is usual to start with low doses and titrate up. After initiation it is important to check the serum urea, electrolytes and creatinine within 7-10 days. A marked rise

Table 5.1 ACE inhibitors*

Indications

Hypertension, left ventricular heart failure and diabetic nephropathy

Cautions

First dose hypotension, renal function should be monitored, hyperkalaemia and aortic stenosis

Contraindications

Hypersensitivity reactions, renal artery stenosis and pregnancy

Side effects

Dry cough, renal impairment, rash, pancreatitis, rhinitis, sore throat, bronchospasm and GI disturbances

Interactions†

Antagonism: NSAIDs, corticosteroids.
Hyperkalaemia: heparins, ciclosporin, K+ sparing diuretics, potassium salts.
Lithium concentration increases

* This table is a generalisation of the prescribing information for ACE inhibitors. You should refer to the data sheet of each individual product before prescribing

† All antihypertensive agents interact with all other antihypertensive agents to cause hypotension; therefore these drugs are not listed. Only significant interactions are listed

in creatinine may indicate a hidden renal artery stenosis, which would prompt stopping the drug. Renal artery stenosis should be suspected in patients with peripheral vascular disease. Each rise in dose as you titrate upwards should be followed by a further blood test, and a rise in creatinine would prompt a reduction in dose. Both ACE inhibitors and ARBs will cause hyperkalaemia. This can be an advantage as they are often co-prescribed with thiazide diuretics, which have the opposite effect, and therefore both drugs cancel each other out. Be very careful if using spironolactone as this also causes hyperkalaemia.

Table 5.2 Angiotensin receptor blockers*

Indications

Hypertension, left ventricular heart failure and diabetic nephropathy

Cautions

Hepatic and renal impairment, aortic stenosis, renal artery stenosis and obstructive hypertrophic cardiomyopathy

Contraindications

Pregnancy and breastfeeding

Side effects

Hyperkalaemia, angioedema, rhinitis, pharyngitis

Interactions†

Antagonism: NSAIDs, corticosteroids.
Hyperkalaemia: heparins, ciclosporin, K+ sparing diuretics, potassium salts.
Lithium concentration increases

* This table is a generalisation of the prescribing information for ARBs. You should refer to the data sheet of each individual product before prescribing

† All antihypertensive agents interact with all other antihypertensive agents to cause hypotension; therefore these drugs are not listed. Only significant interactions are listed

The only major difference between the various ACE inhibitors or ARBs is their duration of action. Captopril, for example, has a short half-life and therefore must be taken twice or thrice daily.

B is for beta-blocker

Sir James Black and others working in the ICI laboratories at Alderley Park developed propranolol in the late 1950s and early 1960s. This drug was the first of many beta-blockers and offered a much more acceptable means of controlling blood pressure than other drugs available at that time. Not only do beta-blockers control blood pressure but they are also of benefit in

---

Box 5.3

Beta-blocker hypertension doses:

- Acebutolol: 200 mg bd to 400 mg bd
- Atenolol: 50 mg od
- Bisoprolol: 5 mg to 20 mg od
- Carvedilol: 12.5 mg to 50 mg od
- Celiprolol: 200 mg to 400 mg od
- Labetalol: 50 mg bd to 600 mg qds*
- Metoprolol: 50 mg to 100 mg bd
- Nadolol: 80 mg to 240 mg od
- Nebivolol: 2.5 mg to 5 mg od
- Oxprenolol: 80 mg od to 160 mg bd
- Pindolol: 15 mg to 45 mg od
- Propranolol: 80 mg to 160 mg bd
- Timolol: 5 mg bd to 20 mg tds

*Liver toxicity risk - requires LFT monitoring

---

patients with dysrhythmias and angina. They have proven efficacy in reducing events following myocardial infarction and benefit people with heart failure.

Like the ACE inhibitors and ARBs, beta-blockers act by reducing the effects of the catecholamines adrenaline and noradrenaline (epinephrine and norepinephrine). Hence there is a lack of synergistic effect with these drugs. As the name implies they work by blocking the beta-adrenoceptors, but they also have some stimulant activity. This stimulant activity varies between the different beta-blockers, as does receptor site specificity and water/fat solubility. Therefore the beta-blockers differ and there is no class effect. This is an important consideration when choosing which one to use.

Beta-blockers reduce heart rate and have a small negative inotropic action, reducing cardiac contractility. They block smooth muscle relaxation in both peripheral blood vessels and bronchi and therefore they cause worsening symptoms in peripheral vascular disease and are contraindicated in asthma. They also cause fatigue and impotence. An important interaction is with the calcium channel blockers diltiazem and verapamil and therefore co-prescribing with these drugs should be avoided in primary care.

The effect on cardiac contractility has caused confusion as to whether or not they are beneficial in heart failure, but overall they are advantageous as long as you choose the right ones - that is, bisoprolol, carvedilol or metoprolol. Remember that in heart failure you must start low and titrate up slowly. My regimen with bisoprolol in heart failure is 1.25, 2.5, 3.75, 5, 7.5 and 10 mg instalments at 1-monthly intervals.

Atenolol is one of the most commonly used beta-blockers, but recent studies have cast doubt on its effectiveness in hypertension. A meta-analysis by Carlberg[3] et al looked at four trials comparing atenolol against placebo and found no significant difference in mortality but fewer cerebrovascular accidents (CVAs) in the atenolol group. Five comparator trials looking at atenolol versus other antihypertensive drugs indicated a higher risk of CHD and CVA events in the atenolol arms.[4] The Carlberg group has recently published a larger meta-analysis in which it attempts to implicate all beta-blockers as inferior antihypertensive agents. The problem with this second paper is that the majority of studies are still atenolol based and none of them include bisoprolol, carvedilol or nebivolol. The group admits that there is a paucity of data for non-atenolol beta-blockers.[5] Further evidence against atenolol has appeared in the early closure of the ASCOT[6] trial blood pressure lowering arm (BPLA) on ethical grounds because of a significantly

Table 5.3 Beta-blockers*

Indications

Hypertension, angina, post-myocardial infarction, arrhythmias, heart failure, thyrotoxicosis, anxiety and migraine

Cautions

Peripheral vascular disease, severe heart failure, phaeochromocytoma (requires concomitant alpha-blocker)

Contraindications

Asthma, profound bradycardia, sick sinus syndrome, second and third degree heart block, cardiogenic shock

Side effects

Bradycardia, bronchospasm, heart block, hypotension, heart failure, peripheral vasoconstriction, fatigue, impotence and GI disturbances

Interactions†

Diltiazem, verapamil, amiodarone, disopyramide, flecainide, procainamide, quinidine. Antagonism: NSAIDs and corticosteroids

* This table is a generalisation of the prescribing information for beta-blockers. You should refer to the data sheet of each individual product before prescribing

† All antihypertensive agents interact with all other antihypertensive agents to cause hypotension; therefore these drugs are not listed. Only significant interactions are listed

higher incidence of secondary endpoint events (fatal/non-fatal CVA, CHD and all-cause mortality) in the atenolol (plus or minus bendroflumethiazide) arm compared with the amlodipine (plus or minus perindopril) arm.

C is for calcium channel blockers

Intracellular calcium exchange regulates vascular smooth muscle and cardiac muscle, causing increased vasodilatation. There are three main types of calcium channel-blocking drugs used in the treatment of hypertension: the dihydropyridines, diltiazem (benzothiazepines) and verapamil (phenylalkylamines). The dihydropyridines are separated into the short-acting drugs such as the nifedipines (also available in a slow-release formulation) and long-acting drugs such as amlodipine and felodipine. There is a simple way of classifying the actions of the three groups in your mind.

- The dihydropyridines are excellent antihypertensives and verapamil is not a very effective antihypertensive

- Verapamil slows the heart, while dihydropyridines speed it up

- Verapamil is very constipating, while the dihydropyridines are not

- Diltiazem is a halfway house in all three considerations *(table 5.4)*

Table 5.4 Effects of calcium channel blockers

	Lowers blood pressure	Effect on heart rate	Causes constipation
Dihydropyridines	▼▼▼	▲	−
Diltiazem	▼▼	▼	+
Verapamil	▼	▼▼	++

Consequently, the dihydropyridines and diltiazem are the only calcium antagonists that should be considered for hypertension control in primary care. The dihydropyridines are most effective and the long-acting formulations have the advantage of being administered only once daily. Diltiazem is of particular use when you also want to control heart rate and a beta-blocker is

Table 5.5 Calcium channel blockers*

Indications

Hypertension, angina and Raynaud's phenomenon

Cautions

Heart failure, pregnancy, breastfeeding

Contraindications

Severe aortic stenosis (diltiazem and verapamil: heart failure, severe bradycardia, sick sinus syndrome and pregnancy)

Side effects

Ankle swelling, headaches, flushing, reflex tachycardia (diltiazem and verapamil: bradycardia, palpitations, constipation and gum hyperplasia)

Interactions†

Antiepileptics (diltiazem and verapamil: beta-blockers, amiodarone, disopyramide, flecainide, procainamide, quinidine)

* This table is a generalisation of the prescribing information for calcium channel blockers. You should refer to the data sheet of each individual product before prescribing

† All antihypertensive agents interact with all other antihypertensive agents to cause hypotension; therefore these drugs are not listed. Only significant interactions are listed

contraindicated (such as in asthma). Calcium channel blockers are very useful in patients with peripheral vascular disease. The single most problematic side effect is swelling of the ankles. There is less ankle oedema if an ACE inhibitor or ARB is already being taken. The theoretical explanation for this is that the arterial dilatation caused by the calcium antagonists is matched by a venous dilatation preventing a tissue pressure difference. Calcium antagonists are negative inotropes and therefore must be used with caution in heart failure.

Box 5.4

Calcium channel blocker hypertension doses:

- Amlodipine: 5 mg to 10 mg od

- Diltiazem: 60 mg tds to 120 mg tds*

- Felodipine: 2.5 mg to 20 mg od

- Isradipine: 1.25 mg to 10 mg bd

- Lacidipine: 2 mg to 6 mg od

- Lercanidipine: 10 mg to 20 mg od

- Nicardipine: 20 mg tds to 30 mg qds*

- Nifedipine LA: 20 mg to 90 mg od

- Nisoldipine: 10 mg to 40 mg od

- Verapamil: 40 mg tds to 120 mg qds

*Once-daily modified-release preparation available

D is for diuretics

There are four types of diuretics: thiazides, thiazide-like diuretics such as chlortalidone or indapamide, loop diuretics such as furosemide or bumetanide, and potassium-sparing diuretics such as amiloride and spironolactone. The indication for the use of spironolactone is different to the general use of diuretics in the ABCD table and is therefore dealt with in the next section (*E is for everything else*).

The thiazides such as bendroflumethiazide and hydrochlorothiazide are the mainstay of blood pressure therapy. Cheap, mostly well tolerated and effective, they are hard to beat. They are particularly useful for elderly and Afro-Caribbean patients.

They work by reducing sodium chloride and water retention, but they are only mildly diuretic. Thiazide diuretics are especially effective when combined with ACE inhibitors, ARBs or beta-blockers, the former two combinations being particularly useful in treating patients with left ventricular hypertrophy. Thiazide-like drugs are very similar, slightly more expensive but in some cases may cause less metabolic disturbance. They are well worth trying if patients cannot tolerate the thiazide diuretics.

Box 5.5

Thiazide/thiazide-like diuretic hypertension doses:

- Bendroflumethiazide: 2.5 mg *mane*

- Chlortalidone: 25 mg to 50 mg *mane*

- Cyclopenthiazide: 250 mcg to 500 mcg *mane*

- Indapamide: 2.5 mg *mane**

- Metolazone: 5 mg *mane*†

- Xipamide: 20 mg *mane*

- Benzthiazide, clopamide, hydrochlorothiazide and hydroflumethiazide are available in various fixed-dose combinations

* Modified release preparation available

† Caution required with concomitant use of loop diuretic

Loop diuretics have very little hypotensive effect and should not be considered as part of the patient's antihypertensive therapy unless the patient has renal impairment or heart failure.

Thiazide diuretics have a fixed-dose reaction, so it is not usually helpful to step up the dose. Most patients will tolerate thiazide diuretics very well. A common side effect, usually experienced shortly after commencing treatment, is a cluster of general malaise, fatigue and light-headed symptoms. This tends to be a temporary experience, so it is well worth warning the patient it may happen and encouraging them to persevere with the treatment if possible.

A common delayed side effect is gout. Pre-existing gout is a relative contra-indication to using these drugs and, if it occurs for the first time as a side effect, you really should stop the thiazide rather than treat the gout with a prophylactic such as allopurinol. Impotence can occur with any hypertensive therapy but is especially likely with thiazides, which is another reason for avoiding their use in young patients if possible. They have a negative effect on glycaemic control but their importance in terms of providing good blood pressure control overrides this in terms of overall benefit to diabetics, and they should still be used. Annual measurement of serum electrolytes is important because these drugs can cause hyponatraemia and hypokalaemia, particularly in the elderly. The combination of a thiazide diuretic and ACE inhibitor usually balances out the effect on potassium.

It is not uncommon to prescribe both a thiazide and a loop diuretic when a patient has hypertension and heart failure. Caution must be exercised when using both as the risk of postural hypotension and salt depletion is far greater. It is also the case that deteriorating heart failure can tip into a low blood pressure state and require less aggressive antihypertensive measures. Apart from regular renal function testing, the best measure of the effects of loop diuretics on the individual are serial measurements of weight. All patients on loop diuretics should have their weight recorded on each visit to the surgery, and the dose of the diuretic should be titrated both up and down on the basis of any weight change.

Table 5.6 Thiazide and thiazide-like diuretics*

Indications

Hypertension, angina and oedema

Cautions

Hyponatraemia, hypokalaemia and severe renal or liver impairment

Contraindications

Gout and Addison's disease

Side effects

Fatigue, impotence, hyponatraemia, hypokalaemia, hypercalcaemia, gout and GI disturbances

Interactions†

Diuretics. NSAIDs cause antagonism and worsening renal function

* This table is a generalisation of the prescribing information for thiazide and thiazide-like diuretics. You should refer to the data sheet of each individual product before prescribing

† All antihypertensive agents interact with all other antihypertensive agents to cause hypotension; therefore these drugs are not listed. Only significant interactions are listed

E is for everything else

Step four of the ABCD Guidelines deals with resistant hypertension and suggests the use of **alpha-blockers** or **spironolactone**.

Alpha-blockers

Alpha-blockers are strange beasts in terms of hypertension treatment. Overall they are too weak to be considered as first line agents, and in fact the alpha-blocker arm of a large recent trial (ALLHAT) was discontinued on ethical grounds for just this reason.[7] They do have a place as additional treatment, especially for men with prostatic hypertrophy, for pregnant women and as fourth-line therapy after A, C and D. Beware the first-dose hypotensive effect, especially in heart failure patients in whom we should, if possible, avoid these drugs.

Aldosterone antagonists

Aldosterone antagonists such as spironolactone are my preferred fourth-line drugs. They are particularly useful in primary aldosteronism/Conn's syndrome (aldosteronism secondary to an adrenal tumour). These conditions should be suspected if the patient has a low potassium and resistant hypertension. Making a diagnosis can be difficult and is sometimes a fruitless process (see Chapter 11). Hence primary aldosteronism/Conn's syndrome is frequently undiagnosed. An alternative, and much more practical, approach is simply to try a low dose of spironolactone (25 mg or even 12.5 mg). There is no advantage in using higher doses. If the patient responds they have primary aldosteronism or Conn's syndrome and should have an abdominal CT scan to exclude an adrenal tumour. A negative scan excludes the diagnosis of Conn's syndrome and indicates a possible ectopic source of aldosterone-secreting tissue, which is likely to elude detection. If the spironolactone works you should obviously continue using it and even consider trying a reduction in other antihypertensive medications. Spironolactone in low doses is safe to use as long as the patient is screened for hyperkalaemia. The patient should be advised to temporarily stop spironolactone if they develop diarrhoea, as it is then that they are at greatest risk of hyperkalaemia.

A new aldosterone antagonist, eplenerone, is now available for the treatment of heart failure, but not yet licensed for hypertension treatment in the UK (similarly, spironolactone is not licensed for this indication in the UK - see Chapters 3 and 8). Eplenerone apparently has the advantage of fewer side effects, including a reduced risk of gynaecomastia.

The only other drugs I would consider using in primary care are the centrally acting antihypertensives. Methyldopa is indicated in pregnancy and is usually instigated by specialists. Moxonidine is a modern central nervous system antihypertensive and the general practitioner with a special interest in hypertension might consider this as part of their armamentarium, but be cautious of its use in heart failure.

We will leave guanethidine, clonidine, sodium nitroprusside and the rest where they belong: consigned to the history books.

Key points

- The ABCD system offers a logical progression in prescribing, using synergistic combinations

- There is controversy about the use of beta-blockers, especially atenolol

- The three main types of calcium channel blockers have very different properties

- Spironolactone should be considered in cases of resistant hypertension

References

1. Williams B, Poulter NR, Brown MJ et al. *J Hum Hypertens* 2004;18(3):139-185

2. Casa JP, Chua W, Loukogeogakis S et al. *Lancet* 2005;366:2026-2033

3. Carlberg B, Samuuelsson O, Lindholm L. Atenolol in hypertension: is it a wise choice? *Lancet* 2004;364:1684-1689

4. Working Party, Medical Research Council. *BMJ* 1992;304:405-412

5. Lindholm L, Carlberg B, Samuelsson O. *Lancet* 2005;366:1545-1553

6. Dahlof B, Sever P, Poulter N et al. *Lancet* 2005;366:895-906

7. The Antihypertensive and Lipid-Lowering treatment to prevent Heart Attack Trial (ALLHAT). *JAMA* 2002;288(23):2998-3007

Chapter 6

Nurse-led hypertension clinics

Learning objectives

After reviewing this chapter you should have a better understanding of:

- The advantages of nurse-led management
- Understanding nurse prescribing legislation
- How a nurse can qualify as a prescriber
- The difference between extended independent and supplementary prescribing
- A description of a supplementary prescribing scheme
- An example of how a clinic can be organised
- Sources of further information

Key words:

Independent prescribing
Supplementary prescribing
Nurse Prescribers' Formulary (NPF)
Nurse Prescribers' Extended Formulary (NPEF)
Extended Formulary for Nurse Prescribers (EFNP)
Clinical management plan
Microsoft Word template

Advantages of nurse-led management

The advantages of nurse-led management are now well recognised in general practice, and old fashioned reluctance by doctors to allow nurses a more active role in medical management should be a thing of the past. In this chapter we will look at the current opportunities for nurse practitioners and practice nurses in prescribing. Further expansion of this role was introduced in May 2006 and the emergence of practice-based commissioning will create an even greater need for nurses to be involved in prescribing for chronic as well as acute conditions.

Nurses are trained to do things properly and not cut corners. Doctors, faced with more to do than time allows, simply cannot dot every 'i' and cross every 't'. Subsequently, they miss out what they see as less important or routine, such as lifestyle advice or the annual blood pressure check. Nurses follow protocols and, on the whole, doctors do not.

Most practices have used nurses to follow-up blood pressure measurement, weigh the patient, advise on diet, check the urine, take the bloods and basically do all the things the doctor never remembers or never seems to have the time to do. In the Whitby practice we have alternated a doctor check and nurse check of patients every 6 months for many years with considerable success.

Now we can take matters a step further. Many practices are allowing nurses to take over the long-term management of hypertension almost entirely. Although doctors remain involved with the initial diagnosis and management planning, the follow-up, uptitration of drugs and steps of adding medication can be performed by the nurse prescriber. This frees up the doctor and saves the patient time too. What is the sense in a nurse finding that a patient is uncontrolled and asking them to make an appointment to see the doctor, when it is clear that an increase in medication is required? In practices where there is no nurse prescriber available they may well simply approach the doctor to change the patient's repeat prescription, but ideally we will all move to nurse prescribing.

Nurse independent prescribing

The first nurse prescribing was the Nurse Prescribers' Formulary (NPF). Used mainly by district nurses and health visitors, this very limited formulary includes few medications and is mainly for wound dressings and appliances. There is an NPF Appendix in the *British National Formulary*. The nurse had to complete a course to be included in this scheme and was then issued with a nurse prescription pad (FP10P in England, marked DISTRICT NURSE/HEALTH VISITOR PRESCRIBER). Many of the products on the NPF are available over the counter and the nurse training courses are no longer available.

An advance on this has been the development of the Nurse Prescribers' Extended Formulary (NPEF) for independent prescribing. These courses for

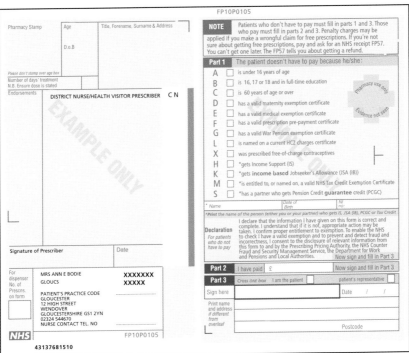

Figure 6.1 District Nurse/Health Visitor FP10P

nurse prescribing (both independent and supplementary prescribing) are available to all registered general nurses (RGNs) and of particular value to nurse practitioners, as well as health visitors, district nurses and community matrons.

Independent prescribing allows the nurse to prescribe all General Sales List Medicines, Pharmacy Medicines and most Prescription Only Medicines. The nurse independent prescriber may prescribe a limited list of controlled drugs; the pharmacist independent prescriber may not.

In order to qualify to do this the nurse must undertake a university-based course. The courses vary, but a typical one might last 6 months and consist of an initial 2-week introductory course followed by 1-day-a-week studying and 1 day training in the practice under the supervision of a doctor, and then

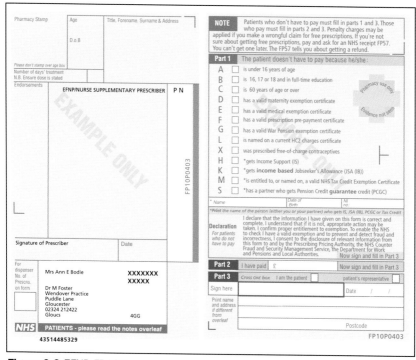

Figure 6.2 EFNP FP10P

a weeklong session at the end. The nurse may also be required to complete an assignment, keep a portfolio, undertake an objective structured clinical examination (OSCE) and sit a written examination. The Nursing and Midwifery Council (NMC) governs the whole process. More information about this can be found at www.nurseprescribing.org.uk. Upon completing the course the nurse is supplied with their own prescription pads, which are purple FP10P forms – the same as for NPF prescribing, except they are marked EFNP/NURSE SUPPLEMENTARY PRESCRIBER. EFNP stands for Extended Formulary for Nurse Prescribers.

Prior to May 2006 an independent nurse prescriber could only prescribe drugs such as antibiotics, antacids, allergy treatments, simple analgesics, steroids and vaccinations. The prescriptions had to relate to specific conditions and the nurse prescriber was much more constrained as regards choice than a medical practitioner. For example, a nurse could prescribe diazepam, but only for palliative care purposes, not for acute anxiety. An up-to-date, comprehensive list of permitted medications and their indications was set out in the Drug Tariff, the Nurse Prescriber Formulary and in the *British National Formulary* NPF appendix. Despite the relaxation of the rules the parameters of prescribing must be agreed with the nurse's manager and employer.

Nurse supplementary prescribing

Supplementary nurse prescribers are not allowed to independently prescribe drugs for hypertension or asthma (except salbutamol). They must follow a clinical management plan individualised for each patient. This management plan must be available on paper or in the patient's computer notes in a set format. The plan must identify the patient, independent prescriber (a doctor in this case) and the supplementary nurse prescribers that it applies to. It will list allergies, the condition being treated and aim of the treatment. It further details the actual drugs used, their indications, dosage titration and specifies at what point the patient should be referred back to the doctor. All guidelines and protocols used must be listed, and the plan must be agreed and signed by the doctor involved. Although this sounds very complicated it is in fact easily done using a Microsoft Word template.

An example of such a clinical management plan template is included in this chapter *(see tables 6.1 and 6.2)*. Each computer on the network should include the template in a desktop folder. The doctor simply opens the template and adds the patient's name, identification number, date of birth and any allergies. Obviously, if the doctor wishes, he or she can also amend more details in the clinical management plan - for example, removing beta-blockers if the patient is asthmatic or thiazides if the patient has gout.

Theoretically the doctor should then print a copy, sign it, ask the nurse supplementary prescribers to sign it (all the nurse prescribers in the practice should be included) and then it should be filed in the patient's paper notes (a legal requirement), although this step may be omitted in a paperless practice. The clinical management plan template can be attached to the patient's computer notes and, because this action is recorded and linked by the computer's audit trail to the password of the doctor performing the action, it is superior to a signature in legal terms. The whole team can now manage this particular patient. The process has to be repeated for each individual patient.

The practice must have a written protocol and formulary for reference by the nurse prescriber. An example of the Whitby Group Practice Protocol is included in *Appendix 2* of this book. For complicated uptitration such as with ACE inhibitors it is best to use a flowchart *(see table 6.2 and figure 6.3, at the end of this chapter)*.

Clearly, individual practices will decide their own parameters and rules for their clinical management plan templates.

In the examples given *(tables 6.1 and 6.2, figure 6.3)*, where generics are not available, I have anonymised the drugs. Choices of which drugs to use are clearly an individual matter for each practice, and I would not seek to tell anyone which specific medication they should have in their formulary. Matters such as the new GMS Contract will influence the blood pressure target, but it is always worth setting your target below the audit target if you want to achieve success.

In the ACE inhibitor flowchart it states that 'if creatinine >150 μmol/l repeat test and inform doctor'. Strictly speaking we should say, 'if creatinine rises by more than 25% repeat the test and inform doctor'. I prefer to keep it simple. Both doctors and nurses are likely to make an error when asked to calculate percentages and a simple 'yes or no' cut-off is less complicated. It is important that the nurse reports this rise, but in many instances I would not get too excited by a small rise in creatinine over 150 μmol/l. The real issue is safe, legal prescribing to cover the nurse's back - hence the need to be pedantic.

Table 6.1 Clinical management plan, example

Name of patient	Patient medication sensitivities/allergies
To be completed by doctor	To be completed by doctor

Patient identification - eg ID number, date of birth
To be completed by doctor

Independent Prescriber(s) (IP)	Supplementary Prescriber(s) (SP)
Name of doctor	Name of nurse

Condition(s) to be treated	Aim of treatment
Hypertension	To achieve BP of 140/85 mmHg or less

Medicines that may be prescribed by SP

Preparation	Indication	Dose schedule	Specific indications for referral back to the IP
To initiate and uptitrate Bendroflumethiazide 2.5 mg od (maintenance dose 2.5 mg) Felodipine 2.5 to 10 mg od Amlodipine 5 to 10 mg od (maintenance dose 5 mg) Lisinopril 2.5 mg od to 20 mg bd (maintenance dose 10 mg) Specific sartan X mg to 4X mg (maintenance dose 2X mg) To uptitrate only Metoprolol 25 to 50 mg bd (maintenance dose 25 mg bd) Bisoprolol 2.5 to 10 mg od (maintenance dose 5 mg)	Reduction in blood pressure	As per Whitby Group Practice protocol, Whitby Group Practice formulary, British National Formulary and British Hypertension Society Guidelines ABCD tables (see below	Failure to achieve target BP with the use of three agents

Table 6.1 Clinical management plan, example (continued)

Guidelines or protocols supporting clinical management plan
- Whitby Group Practice Hypertension Protocol
- Whitby Group Practice Formulary
- *British National Formulary* (BNF)
- BHS Guidelines: Williams B, Poulter NR, Brown MJ et al. *J Hum Hypertens* 2004;18:139-185

Frequency of review and monitoring by

SP	SP and IP
As indicated by response to treatment, but no less than 6 monthly	Annually

Process for reporting adverse events
SP to report to IP and record in records. Notify by yellow card system if indicated

Shared record to be used by IP and SP
Practice computerised record (EMIS)

Agreed by IP(s)   **Date**

Agreed by SP(s)   **Date**

Date agreed with patient/carer

Table 6.2 Prescribing steps (warn all male patients to report impotence)

• Bendroflumethiazide: 2.5 mg maintenance dose 2.5 mg	Warn the patient that they may feel under the weather initially and should try to persevere with treatment Contraindicated in gout
• Metoprolol: 25 mg bd, 50 mg bd (maintenance dose 25 mg bd) • Bisoprolol: 2.5 mg daily, 5 mg daily, 10 mg daily (maintenance dose 5 mg daily)	Doctor initiation only Contraindicated in asthma, COPD, peripheral vascular disease, heart block (patient must have ECG before prescribing) Care required in heart failure
• Felodipine: 2.5 mg daily, 5 mg daily, 10 mg daily	Maintenance dose 5 mg daily for both drugs
• Amlodipine: 5 mg daily, 10 mg daily (for patients with heart failure)	Warn patients regarding swollen ankles
• Lisinopril: 2.5 mg daily, 5 mg daily, 10 mg daily, 20 mg daily, 20 mg bd (maintenance dose 10 mg daily)	(See flowchart) Do not initiate if creatinine is >150 µmol/l. Check U&Es within 2 weeks of initiation and each dose change. If creatinine >150 µmol/l repeat test and inform doctor. If potassium rises above 5.2 mmol/l repeat test and inform doctor. Advise patient to take initial two doses at night. Warn patient about cough. Warn them to report rashes or swollen face within 2 weeks of initiation. Not for patients who are or could get pregnant
• Specific sartan; X mg, 2X mg, 4X mg (maintenance dose 2X mg)	(Same as for lisinopril) Check U&Es within 2 weeks of initiation and each dose change Not for patients who are or could get pregnant

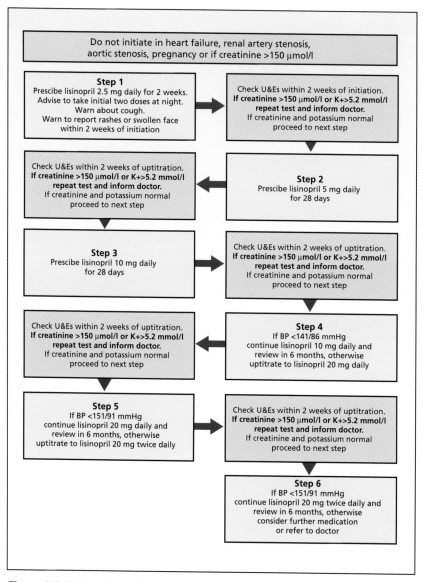

Figure 6.3 Whitby Group Practice flowchart for nurse initiation and uptitration of ACE inhibitors and ARBs

1st May 2006

Restrictions on nurse and pharmacist independent prescribers were relaxed on 1st May 2006. They are now allowed to prescribe most drugs, with some restrictions on controlled drugs, as long as they have personally assessed the patient. They may prescribe off-licence but not unlicensed drugs. Despite these changes the employer is held vicariously liable for the actions of the nurse and must agree the parameters of prescribing. It remains to be seen what attitude the providers of professional indemnity insurance will take. Nurses themselves may be wary of taking on too much responsibility. It is therefore likely that clinical management plans will continue to be seen as a sensible approach and supplementary prescribing might remain popular.

Key points

- Nurse practitioners can take over the majority of hypertension management through independent or supplementary prescribing

- Clinical management plans and practice-based protocols are required as part of the process of supplementary prescribing

- Despite relaxation of restrictions to independent nurse prescribing, working to clinical management plans and protocols is still the wise approach.

Further information

PACT:
www.ppa.org.uk/ppa/info_prescribers_for_pmd_pact.htm

Nurse practitioner UK:
www.nursepractitioner.org.uk/

Northern Ireland:
www.dhsspsni.gov.uk/publications/2004/nurse_prescribing_in_hpss_ni.pdf

Improving Patients' Access to Medicines: A Guide to Implementing Nurse and Pharmacist Independent Prescribing within the NHS in England.
www.dh.gov.uk/PublicationsAndStatistics/Publications/
PublicationsPolicyAndGuidance/PublicationsPolicyAndGuidanceArticle

Chapter 7

Other risk factors

Learning objectives

Hypertension cannot be looked at in isolation. Here we consider the other risk factors both in their cumulative effect and in the case of cholesterol as a single risk factor. We shall look at the latest risk tables and their use in primary prevention. Antithrombotic therapy is considered, as is the diabetic patient. In particular we will look at the second Joint British Society Guidelines published in *Heart*, December 2005.[1]

Key words:

Risk assessment

Absolute risk

Relative risk

Lipids management

Antithrombotic therapy

Diabetes

Primary prevention

Risk tables

Cholesterol as a single risk factor

Global risk assessment

In the hierarchy of cardiovascular risk prediction, high blood pressure is only one factor and by no means does it have the highest predictive value. Some of the highest-ranking predictors of cardiovascular risk are irreversible - for example, pre-existing cardiovascular disease, increasing age, left ventricular hypertrophy and male sex. One of the best indicators of high risk is having a low HDL-C (high-density lipoprotein cholesterol) but there is no evidence that increasing HDL-C improves outcome. High LDL-C (low-density lipoprotein cholesterol) and hypertension are not necessarily such strong predictors but we do know that changing them improves outcome.

Overall no single element gives us absolute predictive power, and nor does changing one factor bring about an especially large change in outcome. Obviously if you have a little bit of every risk factor the cumulative risk outweighs any single factor. Hence the growth of the primary prevention risk prediction industry and the formulation of the risk prevention charts.

Table 7.1 Ranking of predictive factors for the development of CVD in hypertensive patients[2]	
Quantitative factors	**Patient factors**
1. Age	= 1 Age greater than 60 years
2. High-density lipoprotein (HDL)	= 1 Pre-existing cardiovascular disease
3. Glucose	3. Low HDL
4. Low-density lipoprotein (LDL)	4. Diabetes
5. Microalbuminuria	5. Chronic renal failure
6. Creatinine	6. Male sex
7. Systolic BP	7. Familial hypercholesterolaemia
8. Total cholesterol	
9. Diastolic BP	
10. Body Mass Index (BMI)	

This chapter will concentrate on looking at the new Joint British Societies Guidelines (JBS 2) in terms of explaining risk prevention and its various facets.

Joint British Societies Guidelines 2

The first JBS Guidelines, published in 1998, represented the views of four highly influential societies.[3] Namely, the British Cardiac Society, British Hypertension Society, British Hyperlipidaemia Association and the British Diabetic Association. The latter two have now changed their names to HEART UK and Diabetes UK, respectively. These guidelines became a major influence on UK government policy in terms of the National Service Framework for Coronary Heart Disease[4] and the more recent new General Medical Services (nGMS) Contract.[5]

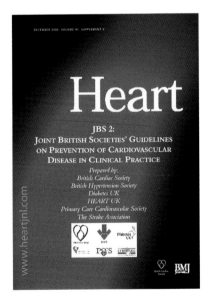

Cover of the *Heart* journal, in which the JBS 2 Guidelines were published

Reproduced with the kind permission of BMJ Publishing Group Ltd

Seven years later we have a new version, JBS 2.[1] This time the original 'gang of four' are joined by the Stroke Association, reflecting the importance of considering total cardiovascular disease risk, and the Primary Care Cardiovascular Society (PCCS), due to the fact that most of this work is performed in general practice.

Much of the hypertension content has already been seen in BHS IV. The full document is published as a supplement to *Heart* and is very long. With more than 50,000 words and 344 references it is unlikely that many primary care doctors or nurses will digest the whole thing.

The new version has taken diabetes out of the primary prevention bracket and treated it as a separate section of its own.

Box 7.1

JBS 2 states that we should focus equally on all people at high risk:

1 People with established atherosclerotic cardiovascular disease*
(CVD)

2 People without established CVD who have an estimated multifactorial CVD risk ≥20% over 10 years of developing atherosclerotic CVD for the first time

3 People with diabetes mellitus (type 1 or 2)

* The category 'established atherosclerotic CVD' includes people with ischaemic heart disease (IHD), peripheral arterial disease (PAD), transient ischaemic attack (TIA) and stroke

---

Apart from the three groups requiring management of their global risk (*box 7.1*), JBS 2 identifies three groups deserving treatment because of 'single risk factors'. The first is rather obvious as it is a standard description of the patient with essential hypertension (*box 7.2*).

Box 7.2

JBS 2, single risk factor 1:

Elevated blood pressure ≥160 mmHg systolic or ≥100 mmHg diastolic, or lesser degrees of blood pressure elevation with target organ damage (140/90 mmHg)

The second group deserving treatment because of single risk factors will be less familiar to most people in that it gives a novel description of the patient with abnormal cholesterol (*box 7.3*). This new definition makes perfect sense as it now takes into account the importance of HDL-C as a marker of high cardiovascular risk and takes us away from just using total cholesterol.

Box 7.3

JBS 2, single risk factor 2:

Elevated total cholesterol:high-density lipoprotein (HDL) ratio $\geq$6.0

In the early drafts of JBS 2 the lipid single risk factor was defined as total cholesterol:HDL-C ratio $\geq$7.0. However, in the final draft, this was changed to the more stringent value of $\geq$6.0. Some controversy may emerge as a result of this decision, and other bodies may wish to adopt the more conservative ratio.

The third group with a single risk factor is more obvious and comprises those with the rare family inherited lipid disorders (*box 7.4*).

Box 7.4

JBS 2, single risk factor 3:

Familial dyslipidaemias, such as familial hypercholesterolaemia or familial combined hyperlipidaemia

---

How the new guidelines work

In the new guidelines CVD risk is calculated, rather than coronary heart disease (CHD) risk, as was the case in JBS 1. The JBS 2 cardiovascular risk charts highlight CVD risks of $\geq$10%, $\geq$20% and $\geq$30% over 10 years. These are equivalent to the old CHD risks of about $\geq$8%, $\geq$15% and $\geq$23%, respectively. The old National Service Framework CHD risk of 30% is the equivalent of a CVD risk of 40%. The NICE statin appraisal released in November 2005 agreed with the JBS 2 proposals and suggests statin treatment for all patients with a CVD risk $\geq$20%.

A bias towards younger populations has been introduced. The age bands are now <50 years, 50 to 59 years and >60 years. At any age less than 50 years the risk is projected to 49 years. At 50-59 years the risk is projected to 59, and everyone 60 and above is considered to be 69 years old. These moves are intended to remove the previous bias of the tables towards older patients receiving treatment and younger patients missing out despite the fact that their total lifetime risk may be exceptionally high.

Two groups of patients are identified as being of even greater risk: those with a strong family history of premature CHD (men <55 years and women <65 years) in a first-degree relative and people from the Indian subcontinent. For both groups, multiply the risk by 1.5 (it's actually slightly higher for Asian people but most of us find it easier to multiply by 1.5 rather than by 1.6!). Furthermore, for Asian people, you should allow for their smaller stature - therefore their normal BMI range is 18 to 23 kg/m^2 and their waist circumference is abnormal if >92 cms in men and >78 cms in women.

Risk is also increased by a factor of 1.3 in people who have fasting triglyceride levels greater than 1.7 mmol/l and increased by a factor of 1.5 in people with impaired glucose tolerance (fasting blood glucose between 6.1 and 6.9 mmol/l). Since the recommendation is to screen with non-fasting samples these two groups may not be identifiable.

The targets set in JBS 2 were first revealed in BHS IV and are described as **optimal targets at which we should aim** and **audit targets by which our performance is judged**. For cholesterol, the 'optimal' total cholesterol target is <4.0 mmol/l and for LDL-C <2.0 mmol/l or a 25% reduction in total cholesterol and a 30% reduction in LDL-C (whichever gets the person to the lowest absolute level). The recommended 'audit standards' are <5.0 mmol/l for total cholesterol or a 25% reduction in total cholesterol, and <3.0 mmol/l for LDL-C or a 30% reduction in LDL-C (whichever gets the person to the lowest absolute level).

When calculating risk it is important to use pretreatment values for blood pressure and lipids. If the pretreatment blood pressure is unknown assume the systolic pressure to be 160 mmHg.

Box 7.5

Key features of JBS 2:

- CVD not CHD risk

- Diabetics are a separate group

- BP ≥160/100 mmHg requires BP control

- TC:HDL ≥6 requires lipid control

- Family history increases risk by 1.5

- South-Asian race increases risk by 1.6

- Ex-smokers must have stopped for 5 years

- Optimal TC target <4.0 mmol/l

- Optimal LDL-C target <2.0 mmol/l

- Audit TC target <5.0 mmol/l

- Audit LDL-C target <3.0 mmol/l

Absolute risk and relative risk

The **risk prediction tables *(figure 7.1)* calculate the individual's absolute risk** of an event occurring. 'Absolute risk' is a projection of risk through time based on all the factors of influence. It compares the individual against the population and gives a percentage chance of something happening to that individual. Once the equation is completed it cannot be improved; it can only get worse.

Professor Paul Durrington of Manchester University is responsible for the JBS 1 and 2 tables and has also created the computer risk models for both guidelines. In the new computer version of the tables, distributed free of charge by the British Heart Foundation to all general practices in the UK, he has added a **relative risk calculator in the form of a thermometer** *(figure 7.2)*. 'Relative risk' is a comparison of the individual against their

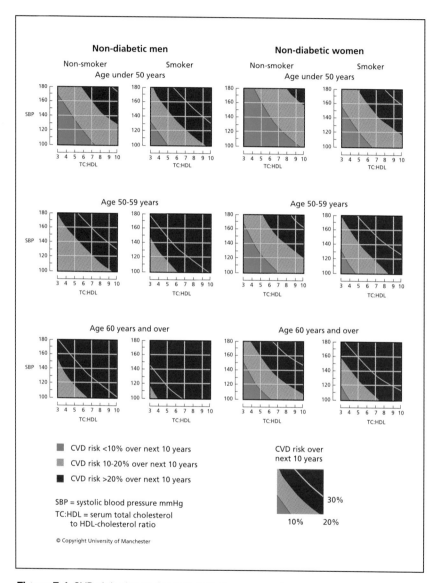

Figure 7.1 CVD risk charts for non-diabetic men and women

Reproduced with the kind permission of Professor Paul Durrington, University of Manchester

peers. It is a ratio of risk rather than a percentage, and gives a range of one to 100. If your risk is less than 50 then you are doing better than people of a similar age and background. You can change your relative risk – hence the relative risk score can be used as a tool to encourage patients to change their lifestyles.

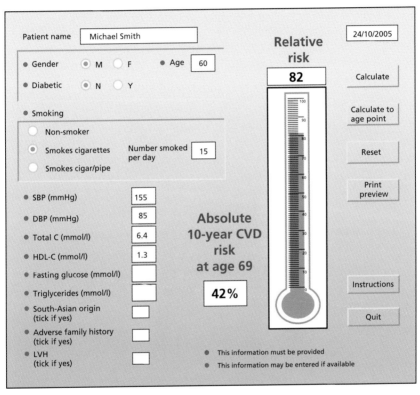

Figure 7.2 Computer cardiovascular risk calculator

Adapted with the kind permission of Professor Paul Durrington, University of Manchester

The doctor or nurse must understand the difference between the two forms of risk calculation if they are to successfully explain the tables to patients.

Metabolic syndrome

The metabolic syndrome, a concept describing the individual who is pre-destined through a combination of genetics and excessive eating to develop both diabetes and CVD, is set to become a more important issue. Originally referred to as syndrome X, or the insulin resistance syndrome, it is spawning a new reason for prescribing prophylactic lipid therapy as well as specific medications to offset its progress. These include the yet-to-be-released cannabinoid receptor blockers, which have already been shown to reduce insulin resistance. Ultimately the most sensible thing would be to encourage people not to become obese.

There are many different diagnostic schedules for metabolic syndrome but JBS 2 sensibly recommends the most straightforward version: the American National Cholesterol Education Program Adult Treatment Panel (NCEP ATP) Guidelines.[6] You must adapt the waistline figures for Asian patients.

Box 7.6

National Cholesterol Education Program (NCEP) metabolic syndrome guidelines:

Diagnosis confirmed if the patient has three out of five conditions:

- Waist circumference >102 cm (men) (Asian men >92 cms) and >88 cm (women) (Asian women >78 cms)

- Blood pressure ≥130/≥85 mmHg

- Fasting glucose ≥6.1 mmol/l

- Serum triglycerides ≥1.7 mmol/l

- HDL-cholesterol <1.0 mmol/l (men) and <1.3 mmol/l (women)

Waist circumference is a better measure of central obesity than body mass index (BMI) and has greater predictive power. It is a horizontal line of cir-cumference from the midway point between the lower rib and the iliac crest. Some people feel this is unreliable because busy doctors will just wrap the measure anywhere around the waist in the hurly-burly of everyday routine work. As if! Alternatively, one can argue that the BMI is an objective measurement, which is therefore destined to remain.

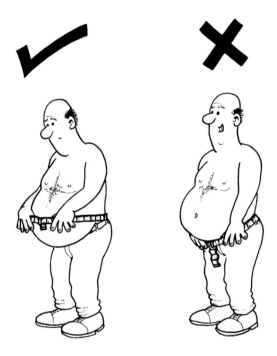

Waist circumference is a better measure of central obesity than body mass index

Lipids management

Dietary cholesterol is not the main source of serum cholesterol. Indeed, less than a quarter of our serum cholesterol has been ingested. Most of it is manufactured in our livers using the fat and protein that we have eaten. This fat and protein is combined to form several lipoproteins, of which the most abundant are LDL-C and HDL-C. LDL-C is a large molecule with a higher proportion of fat than the smaller and denser HDL-C. Although it is probably an oversimplification, we can imagine - and tell our patients - that LDL-C takes fat to the arteries and HDL-C brings it back. This LDL-C liver manufacturing process involves HMG co-reductase, an enzyme inhibited by statins - these drugs are the most effective means of controlling LDL-C. In addition to reducing LDL-C, and therefore total cholesterol, they may in some cases slightly raise HDL-C (by between 2% and 5%), which is probably a good thing - although there is no evidence yet that this reduces morbidity or mortality. Remember that exercise raises HDL quite effectively, and alcohol lowers it. Statins are also believed to have an anti-inflammatory action, which stabilises atheromatous plaques and therefore contributes to their beneficial effects.

Having decided that your patient requires treatment for raised cholesterol, the most likely first step is the prescription of a statin. Do not forget, however, to stress the need to continue a low fat diet, emphasising that all the evidence that statins reduce cardiac endpoints is based on patients who also follow dietary advice.

Your choice of statin will be based on price and efficacy. UK doctors have always tended towards conservative prescribing and therefore used the lowest dose of statins. In the case of simvastatin this was the 10 mg formulation, a dose that will successfully control very few patients. The Heart Protection Study showed us that 40 mg of simvastatin is the optimum dose,[6] but even that amount will control only about 50-60% of your patients. Whichever statin you use there will be an optimum dose - not usually the lowest one. In most cases the statin should be taken in the evening, as this is the time of day when most lipid metabolism takes place. However, long acting statins display little variation in serum concentration and therefore this advice is not required with these drugs. Having established the patient on the optimum dose, you should recheck their cholesterol after 1 to 3 months, depending on the statin you have used. If the patient is still uncontrolled it may be necessary to titrate them to the maximum dose of their statin or change to a stronger statin. In some cases even that will not work and you may need to consider a second drug.

Table 7.2 Common statins*

Statin	Lowest dose	Optimum dose	Maximum dose	How soon to check cholesterol	When to take tablet
Atorvastatin	10 mg	20 mg	80 mg	1-3 months	Any time
Fluvastatin	20 mg	80 mg	80 mg	3 months	Evening
Pravastatin	10 mg	40 mg	40 mg	3 months	Evening
Rosuvastatin	5 mg	10 mg	20/40 mg	1 month	Any time
Simvastatin	10 mg	40 mg	80 mg	3 months	Evening

* This table is a generalisation of the prescribing information for statins. You should refer to the data sheet of each individual product before prescribing

Fibrates have traditionally been our second line drugs. Although the serious statin side effect of rhabdomyolysis is extremely rare it is fatal in 7% of cases, and 60% of rhabdomyolysis cases are due to drug interactions (*see box 7.7*). One of the most common interactions is when statins and fibrates are combined. Therefore many GPs wisely avoid this combination themselves and refer patients needing this step to lipid clinics.

One recent development of note is the introduction of cholesterol absorption inhibitors. As already stated, very little cholesterol is introduced through the diet and therefore you might think that blocking its absorption should not be very effective. It is effective, however, because most of the liver-generated cholesterol is excreted through the biliary system into the intestine and then reabsorbed via a re-uptake mechanism. Cholesterol absorption inhibitors prevent this re-uptake and therefore have a profound effect on serum LDL-C when combined with statins.[7] Because they work in the intestine and are not metabolised in the liver they do not have any negative interaction with statins and are therefore a safe option for combination therapy in primary care.

Box 7.7

Drugs that interact with statins:

- Fibrates, gemfibrozil, nicotinic acid
- HIV protease inhibitors
- Itraconazole, ketoconazole
- Coumarins, warfarin
- Nefazodone
- Ciclosporin
- Digoxin, amiodarone
- Erythromycin, clarithromycin, telithromycin, fucidin
- Protease inhibitors, diltiazem, verapamil, antacids
- Grapefruit juice, Chinese red rice

Apart from statins, fibrates and cholesterol absorption inhibitors, we also have nicotinic acid and omega 3 fatty acids in our armamentarium. Nicotinic acid will lower triglycerides and raise HDL more effectively than statins. Unfortunately, these drugs tend to cause facial flushing, which patients find very irritating, although this is less prevalent with newer formulations. Omega 3 fatty acids have been shown to reduce events post MI and also to lower triglycerides. They do not, however, reduce LDL-C – hence there is no measure of their effect. Patients can theoretically achieve the same benefits by eating lots of oily fish.

Rhabdomyolysis

As already stated, the serious side effect of rhabdomyolysis is very rare. The number needed to harm (NNH) is approximately 1 per 100,000 prescriptions and the number needed to kill (NNK) with a statin rhabdomyolysis is about one in every one million prescriptions.[8] Nonetheless care must be taken to avoid this and, in particular, we must be careful about drug interactions (*see box 7.7*). If a patient complains of muscle aching we should carry out

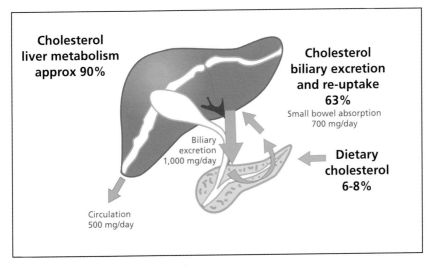

Figure 7.3 Sources of cholesterol

creatinine kinase (CK) estimation. If this is more than three times the upper limit of normal (ULN) we should consider a retest; if it is more than five times the ULN we should stop the statin prescription; and if it is greater than 10 times the ULN we should consider this as a possible myositis. Rhabdomyolysis will typically cause a CK in the 10s of 1,000s mmol/l and there will be myoglobin in the urine. You are very unlikely to ever see a case.

Antithrombotic treatment

The decision to treat people with low dose aspirin comes down to a risk vs benefit calculation. In terms of gastrointestinal bleeds with aspirin, the NNH in 1 year is 248 and the NNK is 2,066.[9] Try comparing that with the statin NNH and NNK! The number needed to treat (NNT) must exceed the NNH before you can recommend this to your patients.

The BHS IV guidelines recommend that **controlled** hypertensives should take aspirin 75 mg, if they are over 50 years of age and also have either target organ damage or diabetes. JBS 2 states that all patients with CVD risk >20% should receive low dose aspirin. Note that the word 'controlled' is highlighted because the risk of haemorrhagic stroke is raised in uncontrolled hypertension.

Obviously some people will not tolerate aspirin and you should consider using clopidogrel in those people.

Warfarin is not indicated in hypertensives or as a primary prevention strategy.

Diabetes and hypertension

The combination of hypertension and diabetes increases the risk of macrovascular disease, microvascular disease and nephropathy. UKPDS proved to us that diabetics were more likely to die from CVD than from any other diabetic complication.[10] The message was stop just being 'sugar doctors' and look at the cholesterol and blood pressure for these patients. As well as UKPDS, hypertension trials such as HOT[11] and HOPE[12] showed us that it was the diabetic patient subsets that derived the greatest benefit in reduction of events with lowering of blood pressure. Even normotensive patients benefited – hence the more aggressive target of 130/80 mmHg for these patients.

ACE inhibitors and ARBs are known to protect diabetics from both micro-albuminuria and nephropathy, as well as helping control blood pressure. Thus they might be considered first line therapy. Diuretics have an adverse effect on glycaemic control, but it has been the opinion of experts that this is outweighed by their benefits in terms of hypertensive control, and the ALLHAT study confirmed this.[13] Calcium channel blockers are apparently quite safe and effective in diabetes, although VALUE did show there were more cases of new-onset diabetes with amlodipine than with valsartan.[14]

ASCOT-BPLA has cast even more doubt on beta-blockers, and especially atenolol,[15] to the point that these drugs really should be considered fourth line in diabetes.

As well as hypertensive management, diabetics require cholesterol control. JBS 2 specifies that all diabetics over 40 years require statins and that those below 40 should have this treatment if they are also hypertensive, if they have nephropathy or retinopathy, if they have total cholesterol over 6 mmol/l, metabolic syndrome or if they have a family history of CVD in a young first degree relative.

The polypill

When the 'polypill' concept was introduced in 2003 it was heralded by the lay media as a major breakthrough that would reduce deaths from heart disease and stroke by 80%.[16] The idea was that a combination of generic drugs could be contained in one pill that would reduce blood pressure and cholesterol while also acting as an antithrombotic *(see box 7.8)*. Folic acid would tackle serum homocysteine. By using generic drugs it would be cheap enough for everyone over 55 years to take it, removing the need for primary prevention assessment and follow-up. Compliance would be good because it was just one pill and, speculating on the available evidence, it was calculated that it would reduce ischaemic heart disease events by 88% (95% CI 84% to 91%) and stroke by 80% (95% CI 71% to 87%).

Nice idea, but there were several reasons why this would always be just a medical fantasy. Mixing the various compounds together would be technically difficult; many individuals would be unable to tolerate one or more of the constituents; individual requirements for more aggressive blood pressure or cholesterol lowering would have to be ignored; and the pharmaceutical licensing requirements as well as legal risks would be insurmountable.

Until such time as pharmacists can technically mix an individual patient's list of medicines into one capsule, the only way to reduce the number of pills required will be by using fixed-dose combinations. In hypertension many such products were made available in previous years but those who taught us in medical school frowned upon their use. Lack of flexibility and increased costs were used as reasons for rejecting fixed-dose combinations. It is perhaps unsurprising therefore that these compounds are little used in the UK at this time. However, this may change for the same reasons the polypill once seemed so attractive. The sheer burden of taking numerous pills is daunting for patients in these days of polypharmacy, with the result that compliance is often reduced. Further, many of the fixed-dose products are now cheaper than the separate components. A change in attitude is required not just by prescribers but also by those who teach medicine.

Box 7.8

Polypill contents:

- Statin
- Thiazide diuretic
- Beta-blocker
- ACE inhibitor
- Folic acid
- Aspirin

Key points

- The decision to treat CVD risk 20% as opposed to CHD risk 30% means many more people will require blood pressure control and statin therapy

- People with diabetes are almost considered as a secondary prevention group

- Low HDL-C is one of the best predictors of risk

- People with a TC:HDL ratio of ≥ 6.0 will be a novel consideration for many practitioners

- Family history of CVD and having an Indian ethnic origin increases the risk of developing CVD by 1.5 times

- An understanding of the difference between absolute and relative risk is vitally important

- The new risk tables have three age bands and are skewed towards including more young patients in the treatment group

References

1. Joint British Societies. *Heart* 2005;91(suppl V):v1-v52

2. Domenech M, Sobrino J, Plana J. Presented at ESH 2005, Milan: Poster P2.109

3. Wood DA, Durrington P, Poulter N et al. *Heart* 1998;80:S1-S29

4. National Service Framework for Coronary Heart Disease. Modern standards and service models. London: Department of Health, March 2000: www.dh.gov.uk/PolicyAndGuidance/HealthAndSocialCareTopics/CoronaryHeartDisease

5. www.dh.gov.uk/PolicyAndGuidance/OrganisationPolicy/PrimaryCare/PrimaryCareContracting

6. Third Report of the Expert Panel on Detecting, Evaluation and Treatment of High Blood Cholesterol in Adults (Adult Treatment Panel III). Executive Summary available at: www.nhibi.nih.gov/guidelines/cholesterol/

7. Heart Protection Study Collaborative Group. *Lancet* 2002;360:7-22

8. Thompson PD, Clarkson P, Karas RH et al. *JAMA* 2003;289:1681-1690

9. Derry S, Loke YK. *BMJ* 2000;321(7270):1183-1187

10. UK Prospective Diabetes Study Group. *BMJ* 1998;317(7160):703-713

11. Hansson L, Zanchetti A, Carruthers SG et al. *Lancet* 1998; 351(9118):1755-1762

12. The Heart Outcomes Prevention Evaluation Study Investigators. *New Engl J Med 20*00;342:145-153

13. The Antihypertensive and Lipid-Lowering Treatment to Prevent Heart Attack Trial (ALLHAT). *JAMA* 2002;288(23):2998-3007

14. Julius S, Kjeldsen SE, Weber M et al. *Lancet* 2004;363:2022-2031

15. Dahlof B, Sever P, Poulter N et al. *Lancet* 2005;366:895-906

16. Wald NJ. Law MR. *BMJ* 2003;326(7404):1419

Chapter **8**

Guidelines

Learning objectives

In this chapter we will look at the advantages and disadvantages of using national or local guidelines, with particular reference to the NICE Guidelines on hypertension. Can or should your local health organisation strictly tell a practice what to do? The development of a practice protocol and formulary will also be explained.

Key words:

Protocol

GOBSAT

British Hypertension Society

National Institute of Clinical Excellence

Scottish Intercollegiate Guidelines Network

Anglo-Scandinavian Cardiac Outcome Trial

Guidelines and protocols

A guideline provides guiding principles that direct action, either official or unofficial, while a protocol sets out rules, codes of behaviour, etiquette and convention. In other words guidelines are the softer option, whereas protocols are more directive, strict and, subsequently, less popular (when sent from above)! We can all do with a little help and advice but we do not necessarily like being told what to do. It is a generalisation, but doctors are less likely to accept direction and nurses tend to welcome advice; we were trained in different ways and have differing philosophies in this regard.

My personal feeling is that organisations such as primary care practices benefit from rules as long as they are rules in which the organisation has a say. Hence my preference is for the development of local protocols based on national guidelines. A local protocol might be solely practice based or produced by the local primary care organisation (PCO) but, whichever it is, the people expected to comply with the document must be given an oppor-tunity to say whether or not they accept the principles in the protocol. Where, as has happened, a PCO directs practices without consultation this should be resisted, because in the final analysis such a protocol is unenforceable over a group of independent practitioners.

The practice I work in is large. We have a regular turnover of new partners; we use locums; we have four new registrars each year, two nurse practitioners, six practice nurses and four healthcare assistants. Over a 10-year period there will be nearly 100 different clinical personnel involved. Considered in the same light, a PCO will have a workforce of over 1,000. To get everyone working to the same agenda and 'singing from the same songsheet', we need written protocols.

Using national guidelines for local policy is fraught with problems. Which guideline do you use? How can you introduce local accountability and ownership? How do you adapt it to local variations in resources? In partic-ular, how do you get people to read national guidelines when they are invari-ably very long, boring and more effective at inducing sleep than temazepam? The answer is: 'you don't; you produce a short, local protocol'.

National guidelines

We have guidelines from societies and from Government approved bodies and, while they all claim to be evidence based, there will always be an element of personal opinion in the final draft. GOBSAT (**G**ood **O**ld **B**oys **S**itting **A**round **T**alking) is one way of describing personal opinion! Everyone has their own perspective or bias, and it is important that this is recognised.

The most influential hypertension guidelines in the UK are probably those of the British Hypertension Society (BHS). This is basically a self-appointed, autonomous club of doctors who are interested in the subject. They are mainly secondary care based or academics. In most cases their livelihoods depend to some extent on the existence and importance of the condition. Nonetheless, I feel that they are a trustworthy lot and their guidelines are excellent. (I am not a member!) That having been said, the first two guidelines they produced had little or no input from primary care. They did, however, consult GPs for the third guideline, and the most recent guidelines include a GP author, Dr Mark Davis from Leeds.

The National Institute of Clinical Excellence (NICE) Guidelines (CG18: *Hypertension [persistently high blood pressure] in adults*) are controversial.[1] NICE is a Government body and the assumption is that it is out to save money. This is not entirely fair, because the review panel consisted of independent people, mostly GPs from the North East of England and one senior member of the BHS, Professor Bryan Williams. Although it advised NICE on the evidence the panel did not have control of the final outcome.

The controversy was the recommendation that all patients should be initiated on thiazide diuretics, then a beta-blocker and then a calcium channel blocker, unless the patient was at risk of developing diabetes. Then an ACE inhibitor or angiotensin receptor blocker (ARB) should be used first line.

Subsequently it was recognised that the NICE Guidelines had sown confusion. The problem was the remit given to the panel. It was not asked to produce a general hypertension guideline but, more specifically, a guideline for primary care patients with uncomplicated raised blood pressure and no

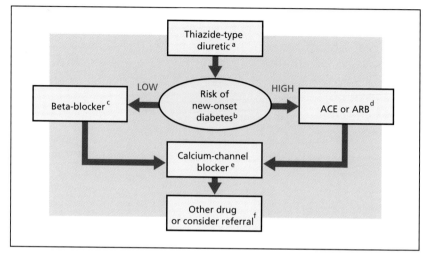

Figure 8.1 The controversial NICE treatment recommendations

comorbidities. Such patients do not have diabetes, ischaemic heart disease, left ventricular hypertrophy or any of the other compelling reasons that would lead the physician to consider using an ACE inhibitor or ARB. Furthermore, the panel did not exclude the use of ACE inhibitors or ARBs in patients without risk of new-onset diabetes; indeed, it suggested these agents as fourth-line drugs. However, *figure 8.1* shows this step described as 'other drug or consider referral', which caused more confusion.

Box 8.1

The original NICE Guidelines excluded many patients:

'This guideline does not address screening for hypertension, management of hypertension in pregnancy or the specialist management of secondary hypertension (where renal or pulmonary disease, endocrine complications or other disease underlie raised blood pressure). Patients with existing coronary heart disease or diabetes should be managed in line with current national guidance for these conditions'

As a result of this confusion and the evidence emerging from the ASCOT-BPLA study on atenolol (see the section later in this chapter), NICE decided to revise its guidance algorithm. Therefore the National Collaborating Centre for Chronic Conditions (NCC-CC), based at the Royal College of Physicians, was commissioned by NICE to update the pharmacological interventions section of the guideline. The NCC-CC convened a small panel of experts representing NICE and the BHS and including a GP member and nurse member of the Primary Care Cardiovascular Society (PCCS). This group produced the new treatment algorithm *shown in figure 8.2, below*, which is evidence based, practical, less controversial and very different from the original guideline algorithm. In essence it is similar to the ABCD table, but without the 'B' step.

This all makes sense, but note that spironolactone, which I have championed in this book, is not mentioned. The reason for this is that there is no evidence base for spironolactone, and nor is it licensed for use in hypertension. It is

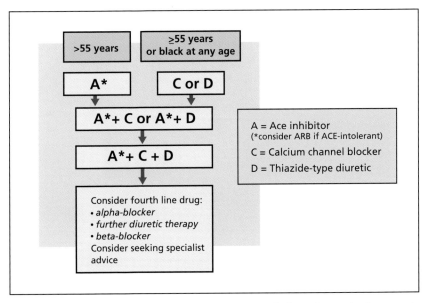

Figure 8.2 The updated NICE treatment recommendations for newly diagnosed hypertension

basically considered as something a specialist would prescribe. I feel this is a pity. The reason spironolactone has no evidence or licence is because it is a generic drug and therefore no industry funds are available to pay for that evidence. Herein lies a fundamental weakness of evidence-based medicine: just because there is no evidence does not mean the hypothesis is untrue.

The danger in using spironolactone is that of failure to carry out long-term follow-up. The problem with a specialist recommendation being the basis of initiation is that invariably the specialist does not carry out the long-term follow up; the primary care team do. This seems an illogical state of affairs.

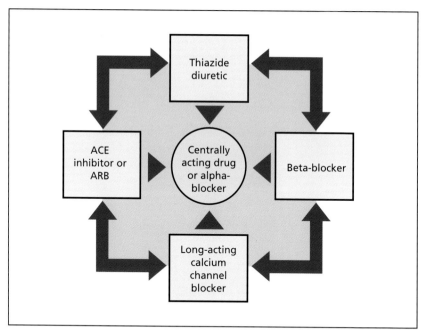

Figure 8.3 The Birmingham System
Start therapy at any square and use add-on therapy on either side as shown by the arrows. Drugs in adjacent squares have additive antihypertensive effects, complementary actions, and are usually well tolerated. Multiple combinations may be required

Less controversial than NICE and better accepted, particularly in Scotland, are the Scottish Intercollegiate Guidelines Network (SIGN) Guidelines.[2] First established in 1993, these are excellent evidence-based guidelines that have been compiled by a broad range of people and, in particular, with strong representation from primary care. There is no specific general hypertension guideline, but the *Hypertension in older people*, Publication No 49, published in January 2001, is pretty much a general guideline and is intended for anyone over the age of 60 years. Unlike NICE, SIGN is much less proscriptive about prescribing and promotes tailored therapy in the main. When combining drugs, SIGN recommends following the Birmingham System. This, like the BHS ABCD approach, allows for the logical addition of drugs in a synergistic manner (*see figure 8.3*).

The second Joint British Society Guidelines (JBS 2) are largely based on the British Hypertension Society's Fourth Guidelines (BHS IV) and include new risk assessment tables (*see Chapter 7*). The original JBS Guidelines, published in 1998, became the basis of the National Service Framework (NSF) for Coronary Heart Disease, and subsequently much of the new General Medical Services (nGMS) Contract was also based on these recommendations. It is likely that the JBS 2 will be equally as influential. Importantly, the new guidelines now incorporate direct influence from primary care, as the Primary Care Cardiovascular Society was one of the six societies involved.

Local protocols

As already stated, local protocols are superior to national ones because the people using them have ownership. They can be adapted to local resources and the people responsible for drafting them are readily accessible.

Mao Tse-Tung said that the longest march starts with a single step and, equally, if you do not have any practice protocols you can start by just putting a few lines on a single sheet of paper. The Whitby Group Practice Hypertension and Lipid Protocols (*see Appendices 2 and 3*) started that way over 15 years ago. We simply stated some desirable aims in terms of whom we wanted to treat and how we wanted to achieve this. Successive redrafts have resulted in the documents printed in this book. While a local protocol should be based on evidence and preferably relate to at least one national guideline, you can put in your own ideas and in particular you can make some of the more idealistic attitudes of the national guidelines more pragmatic. Regular updates are important and every now and then a complete rewrite is required. One or two people should take prime responsibility for each protocol but everyone involved should approve it before completion. I call it a 'protocol' because, at the local level, you should be able to accept it as your own rulebook and use it to set your own consistent standard.

Such a protocol should be the basis for audit and results of local audits should be taken into account when redrafting the protocol. We publish all our protocols on our practice Intranet and also produce a loose-leaf book for internal use. You will note from *Appendix 2* that the protocol also contains our formulary selections. In this, I have included the generic name where available but anonymised the drugs that are available only as brands. Clearly the choice of drugs is a local issue and can be based on local financial considerations. Our choice of drugs changes frequently.

PCO-based protocols can be more difficult to achieve, because there are so many more people to consult. I would not accept a protocol in which I was not given the opportunity to make a comment or contribution.

Much in the Whitby Group Practice Protocols is based on national guidance or is explained in various sections of this book. The protocols are designed to be simple to refer to – this explains why each forms a series of lists. If anyone in the practice has a query about the protocol or does not understand it, they simply have to ask someone else to explain matters. If the explanation does not work we change the protocol.

Has ASCOT put the 'hype' into hypertension?

ASCOT (the Anglo Scandinavian Cardiac Outcome Trial)[3] is the most recent large trial in hypertension and deserves some special attention. The blood pressure-lowering arm (BPLA) was designed to answer the question whether modern antihypertensive drugs have some advantage over older agents and, in particular, if the disappointing CHD outcomes of older trials could be explained by such differences. The trial was well designed and well run: in essence 19,257 patients were randomised into two groups receiving, in one arm, atenolol followed by bendroflumethiazide and, in the other, amlodipine followed by perindopril. The patients were aged 40 to 79 years and the design was open label prescribing with blinded endpoints. This was not a primary prevention trial because the patients had to have at least three cardiovascular risk factors, as listed in *box 8.2*. The ethics committee stopped the trial early, after a median of 5.5 years, because of the excess events in the atenolol arm.

Box 8.2

ASCOT participants had three or more CVD risk factors:

- Left ventricular hypertrophy
- Type 2 diabetes
- Peripheral artery disease
- Stroke/TIA
- Male sex
- Age >55 years
- Microalbuminuria/proteinuria
- Smoker
- Total cholesterol:HDL >6 mmol/l
- Family history of premature CHD

Exclusions included:

- Past medical history of MI
- Angina
- CVA within 3 months
- Triglycerides >4.5 mmol/l
- Heart failure
- Uncontrolled arrhythmia

The trial did not reveal statistically significant differences between treatments in terms of the primary endpoints of fatal CHD or non-fatal MI, although there were 35 more deaths in the atenolol arm. It did reveal statistically significant differences favouring amlodipine for the secondary endpoints of total coronary events (13%), total cardiovascular events (16%), all-cause mortality (11%), cardiovascular mortality (24%) and all strokes (23%).

So what did ASCOT tell us?

The most important message was that, by using a well-structured approach and two or more medications in 78% of patients, we could reduce mean population blood pressure from 164/95 mmHg to 137/78 mmHg. The target blood pressures of <130/80 mmHg in diabetics and <140/90 mmHg in everyone else were achieved in 53% of patients (60% of those without diabetes). The newer drugs amlodipine and perindopril were associated with fewer cardiac events and less new-onset diabetes. This validates the BHS's A(B)CD approach (see Chapter 7).

The ALLHAT study[4] suggested that there was no difference between thiazides, calcium channel blockers and ACE inhibitors. However, it did not measure the effect of atenolol, as this agent was the second-line drug for all study participants. Hence we can conclude that atenolol may not be the best drug to use for the treatment of non-CHD-associated hypertension.

As in the VALUE study,[5] the amlodipine arm may have outperformed the comparator drug because blood pressure control was achieved faster. This may suggest that aggressive early therapy is preferable for all hypertensive patients.

The ethics committee stopped the lipid-lowering arm of the trial after only 18 months because the events in the non-treatment arm were excessively disproportionate to those in the treatment arm. This arm of the trial told us that people with hypertension and three other cardiovascular risk factors do benefit from statin therapy.

What ASCOT did not tell us

This trial did not reach its primary endpoints and so there is no proof that calcium channel blockers and ACE inhibitors are superior to thiazides as regards preventing mortality. An attempt to make more of the results by serial mean matching (which basically means you match patients with similar demographics/characteristics and the same reduction in blood pressure in order to remove the blood pressure-lowering effect on their outcome) may be taking statistical manipulation too far.

It was also claimed that the calcium channel blocker, ACE inhibitor and statin caused a 48% reduction in relative risk compared with the beta-blocker, thiazide and no statin. This may be misleading as in effect the study was comparing use of a statin against placebo (which makes up the majority of the difference) and mixing in the difference in the contributions of the blood pressure medications (which was only small).

There was a great deal of 'lay' or general media attention after the final trial results were announced. This led some critics to claim that ASCOT was overhyped. This was regrettable as it was an important trial that has advanced our knowledge of hypertension and cholesterol management.

Key points

- Guidelines advise on principles and protocols indicate rules

- The best protocols are written locally, based on national guidelines

- Guidelines such as NICE can cause confusion if people do not understand the original remit

- ASCOT told us that aggressive treatment of blood pressure and cholesterol is effective in reducing cardiovascular events

References

1. Available at: www.nice.org.uk/page.aspx?o=cg

2. Available at: www.sign.ac.uk/guidelines/published/numlist.html

3. Dahlof B, Sever P, Poulter N et al. *Lancet* 2005;366:895-906

4. The Antihypertensive and Lipid-Lowering Treatment to Prevent Heart Attack Trial (ALLHAT). *JAMA* 2002;288(23):2998-3007

5. Julius S, Kjeldsen SE, Weber M et al. *Lancet* 2004;363:2022-2231

Chapter 9

Blood pressure control in obstetrics, anaesthetics, nephrology and stroke

Learning objectives

Here we look at four situations where the treatment of blood pressure is very different from the straightforward management generally seen in primary care. Hypertension in obstetrics, anaesthetics and nephrology is always a matter for specialist care and, increasingly, this is becoming the case in stroke too. However, care is often shared, so an understanding of the principles of treatment is useful. In the case of obstetric hypertension we consider how best to manage the patient after she has delivered. We will look at the concept of perioperative hypertension in anaesthesia. Renal disease requires the use of loop diuretics as antihypertensive agents. Stroke may be the first presentation of a hypertensive illness and requires careful introduction of therapies.

Key words:

Hypertension of pregnancy

Pre-eclampsia

Perioperative hypertension

Chronic kidney disease

Antithrombotics

Management of hypertension in pregnancy

It is normal for blood pressure to fall during pregnancy because of reduced peripheral vascular resistance. Most hypertensive pregnant patients have pre-eclampsia, a condition characterised by having a diastolic blood pressure greater than 90 mmHg at more than 20 weeks' gestation, as well as proteinuria. A diastolic blood pressure of greater than 110 mmHg is considered severe.

Some patients may have had an undetected hypertension prior to pregnancy - if they have high blood pressure without proteinuria before 20 weeks' gestation, they may be considered to have pre-existing hypertension. Young women with pre-existing hypertension are more likely to have a renal condition as the primary cause. Hence renal function testing is important.

If hypertension is untreated there is a high risk of developing the life threatening condition of eclampsia and this, rather than long-term cardiovascular disease (CVD), is the immediate concern. A cardiovascular risk score assessment would be inappropriate, but if it were to be performed these patients would have a low score. Long term, women who suffer pre-eclampsia have a higher risk of CVD in later life, but that risk is reduced for women whose subsequent pregnancies are normotensive.[1]

Box 9.1

Obstetric hypertension:

- <20 weeks = hypertension of pregnancy
  ≥20 weeks = pre-eclampsia

- Mild hypertension treatment: rest/drugs

- Severe hypertension treatment: delivery

- After delivery the patient often does not require ongoing drug treatment

---

The management of hypertension in pregnancy, when mild, is based on rest and using drugs that are not toxic to the fetus. When severe, the pregnancy should be ended as soon as possible, by delivery or termination.

Usually the obstetricians will take responsibility for the key management decisions, based on national or regional guidelines. If there is a further complication such as renal or structural cardiac disease, the relevant medical specialist will also become involved.

The timing of interventions is of crucial importance and therefore very frequent antenatal monitoring is required. Obstetric services are becoming increasingly day-care orientated. Hence the patient may go home at night, following rest accompanied by maternal and fetal monitoring in the day unit.

Methyldopa and labetalol are the most common first-line drugs, with nifedipine as second line. ACE inhibitors and angiotensin receptor blockers (ARBs) are absolutely contraindicated in pregnancy because of their effect on fetal growth.

Table 9.1 Patients at high risk of eclampsia[2]
Severe hypertension:
>170/110 mmHg with proteinuria + (1 g)
OR moderate hypertension:
>140/90 mmHg with proteinuria ++ (3 g)
PLUS
any alarm symptoms or signs: headache, visual disturbance, epigastric pain, clonus, papilloedema, liver tenderness, platelet count <100x10^9/l, ALT >50 iu/l

Where there is a high risk of eclampsia delivery will be undertaken – usually by lower segment caesarean section – whether the fetus is viable or not. Termination may be the only choice in the early cases. In established eclampsia intravenous infusions of magnesium sulphate are used both as prophylaxis and as treatment for convulsions, but should be introduced only

Table 9.2 Drugs used in hypertension of pregnancy

Methyldopa

Dose 250 mg bd to 1 g tds

Contraindicated in depression, active liver disease, phaeochromocytoma and porphyria

Labetalol

Dose 100 mg bd to 400 mg bd

Contraindicated in asthma, heart block, uncontrolled heart failure.

Risk of liver damage, therefore liver function tests required for monitoring

Long-acting nifedipine (unlicensed use)

Dose 20 mg od to 90 mg od

Contraindicated in aortic stenosis, post MI and porphyria

Hydralazine

Dose 25 mg bd to 50 mg bd. IV in hypertensive crisis

Contraindicated in systemic lupus erythematosus, severe tachycardia, cor pulmonale, dissecting aneurysm

Thiazides

Last resort

ACE inhibitors and ARBs

Totally contraindicated

with caution in the oliguric patient. Ultimately, diazepam or general anaesthesia may be required to stop convulsions in some women.

Primary care involvement revolves around diagnosis, referral, facilitation of prescriptions and assistance with monitoring during the pregnancy. In the postpartum period, however, the future management may become solely the charge of the GP. Most women with pre-eclampsia will successfully stop their medication, but a gradual reduction of dose together with frequent monitoring of blood pressure is required. If medication is completely stopped, the combined oral contraceptive pill should be avoided and annual checks of blood pressure should be considered. Hormone replacement therapy does not cause hypertension.

Counselling on and education about future pregnancies should include the need to plan matters as well as early antenatal care. Pre-eclampsia is less likely in future pregnancies if the woman has the same partner as in the index event.

Women with pre-existing hypertension will need to continue medication and it would be sensible to avoid ACE inhibitors and ARBs unless sterilisation has been performed. When judging the need for continued medication in the postnatal period you should now consider the CVD risk calculation - in many cases this will be very low.

Anaesthesia and perioperative raised blood pressure.

Here we need to understand two different philosophical concepts of raised blood pressure.

Anaesthetists look at blood pressure from a different point of view to physicians. They are experts in the acute dynamic changes in blood pressure. Their concern is what happens in the hours and days during and after the operation. Perioperative morbidity and mortality is measured up to 30 days after the operation. **Anaesthetists are concerned with perioperatively raised blood pressure.**

Primary and secondary care physicians are interested in the long-term effects of chronic hypertension.

These are not comparable conditions.

Table 9.3 Differences in the management of blood pressure			
(✔ = normal BP)	Home	Clinic	Hospital
Normotensive	✔	✔	✔
Perioperative high BP	✔	✔	✘
White coat high BP	✔	✘	✘
Hypertensive	✘	✘	✘

The patient arriving in hospital for an anaesthetic will be nervous, and blood pressure measurement may reveal an extreme of white coat hypertension. Table 3 shows what I describe as another stage between normotension and white coat hypertension: namely, perioperative hypertension. This is one of the most common reasons for operations being postponed or cancelled. The patient may be sent back to the GP to get the blood pressure 'sorted out' but then have normal blood pressure in the surgery. In such cases the anaesthetists need to be informed of the situation. They may still require the patient to have treatment because they take their evidence from short-term trials showing that perioperative cardiovascular risk relates to the highest recorded blood pressure, not the resting blood pressure. The treatment is usually with beta-blockers because anaesthetists also relate risk to the 'rate-pressure product' (pulse rate multiplied by the diastolic blood pressure). This treatment can be short term, starting a week or so before surgery and stopping shortly afterwards, an approach that is similar to that for woman with pre-eclampsia. The important thing is that these patients are not labelled as hypertensive for the rest of their lives because of this temporary situation.

Some patients may have a previously undiagnosed essential hypertension. Those patients should not be diagnosed solely on the hospital measurements. Instead, carry out at least three measurements, as described earlier in this book (*see Chapter 1*). They may need a longer period of treatment before returning for surgery because circulating volumes require some time to adjust to treatment.

Increasingly, patients attend preassessment clinics before undergoing anaesthesia. This is a much better environment to measure blood pressure accurately. Nonetheless it is only one measurement, and in a clinical setting, and therefore is not something upon which to base a lifetime of drug therapy. There are also conflicting policies in differing hospital departments. In a survey of the cancellation rates for hypertensive patients undergoing anaesthesia and elective surgery, undertaken by way of a questionnaire of anaesthetic departments in Southwest England, there was wide variation in blood pressure guidelines.[3] Most departments still used the American Joint National Committee's stage III cut-off point of diastolic blood pressure 110 mmHg, and there was often no recommendation for systolic blood pressure.

Obviously if the surgery is urgent a compromise arrangement is required. In the emergency situation the anaesthetist can bring the patient's blood pressure under control using standard oral drugs as well as various intravenous agents. The vasodilator sodium nitroprusside works by acting like nitric oxide on vascular smooth muscle. Adrenergic blockade can be achieved by using the beta-blocker esmolol, the alpha-blocker phentolamine or a combination in the form of labetalol.

To quote Professor Prys-Roberts, a leading authority on hypertension in anaesthesia and hypertension, *'the only justification for postponing surgery is to... improve the patient's medical condition'*.[4]

Renal disease and hypertension

Patients with hypertension and severe chronic kidney disease, as defined by an eGFR of less than 30, should be referred to a renal physician for advice. In mild to moderate renal failure they may prefer that we look after the hypertension and, as far as this is concerned, the basic rule is get as low as is practical to protect the kidney. Any patient with blood pressure greater than 140/90 mmHg should be treated to the treatment target of 130/75 mmHg, or even lower if proteinuria exceeds 1 g per 24 hours. These low pressures are known to reduce the progression of renal disease. A past history of hypertension of pregnancy is quite frequently seen in patients with chronic kidney disease (CKD).

Box 9.2

Renal patients require:

- Very low blood pressure
- Loop diuretics
- ACE inhibitors or ARBs
- Close monitoring of renal function (eGFR) and weight

Diuretics are usually used first choice because sodium and water retention is a key part of the problem due to compensatory mechanisms coming into play. The diseased kidneys can be resistant to the effect of thiazides, so high-dose loop diuretics are necessary. This is one situation where loop diuretics will have a significant effect on blood pressure reduction.

The most useful serial measurement apart from renal function is patient weight, as this indicates the amount of water retention and will allow both up- and down-titration of diuretics. Estimated glomerular filtration rate (eGFR) is recommended as superior to serum creatinine in the *National Service Framework for Renal Services* (*see Chapter 7*). Think of eGFR as being equal to the percentage of renal function remaining.

ACE inhibitors have an additive protective element in renal disease and are often the preferred second-line therapy. However, they are contraindicated in cases of renal artery stenosis. ARBs will provide similar benefit to ACE inhibitors. It is important to continue ACE inhibitors and ARBs even if eGFR falls by up to 20% or creatinine increases by up to 30%. Dihydropyridine calcium channel blockers are not renoprotective.

Be careful with metformin, which must be avoided in stage 4 disease. At CKD stage 4 we should also reduce the dose of allopurinol and minimise the use of NSAIDs. Most acute-on-chronic problems occur with multiple insults when the patient is on ACE inhibitors, loop diuretics and NSAIDs and then gets sepsis and volume depletion. So take great care with the acutely sick CKD patient.

Table 9.4 Stages of chronic kidney disease		
Stage	**eGFR**	**Description**
1	90+	Normal kidney function but urine or other abnormalities point to kidney disease
2	60-89	Mildly reduced kidney function; urine or other abnormalities point to kidney disease
3	30-59	Moderately reduced kidney function
4	15-29	Severely reduced kidney function
5	14 or less	Very severe, or endstage kidney failure

The importance of CKD and hypertension was highlighted by the changes made to the nGMS Quality Outcome Framework (QOF) in the 2006 update. Twenty-seven additional points became available for CKD and blood pressure treatment (table 9.5).

Stroke and hypertension

Stroke may be the first presentation of hypertension and this is particularly sad in the patient who has no record of blood pressure measurement for many years or, worse still, the patient who defaulted on treatment. The person with any form of stroke deserves immediate hospital assessment and treatment. The worst cases may need to be considered for thrombolysis. The mildest transient ischaemic attacks (TIA, less than 24-hour duration) are at high risk of recurrence and need accurate diagnosis, consideration of blood pressure treatment and ongoing antithrombotic treatment.

Table 9.5 Additional QOF points available for the treatment of CKD and hypertension

Indicator		Points	Maximum threshold
CKD 1	The practice can produce a register of patients aged 18 years and over with CKD stage 3-5	6	
CKD 2	The percentage of patients on the CKD register whose notes have a record of blood pressure in the previous 15 months	6	90%
CKD 3	The percentage of patients on the CKD register in whom the last blood pressure reading, measured in the last 15 months, is 140/85 mmHg or less	11	70%
CKD 4	The percentage of patients on the CKD register treated with an ACE inhibitor or ARB, unless contraindicated	4	80%

Box 9.3

Stroke victims require:

- Specialist assessment
- Careful blood pressure control
- Antithrombotics after BP control
- Statin therapy

It is very important not to rush in with excessive blood pressure-lowering medication, as this may be counterproductive. The pressure can be particularly elevated post stroke and in the weeks after the event will reduce naturally. Therefore a 'happy medium' approach is warranted and we should tackle the hypertension gently. It is very important that antithrombotic therapy such as aspirin (with or without dipyridamole) or clopidogrel is not started until the precise diagnosis is made and that the blood pressure is controlled, as otherwise a catastrophic haemorrhage may result. Warfarin is the preferred agent in atrial fibrillation or recurrent strokes.

In the long term, stroke patients have cardiovascular disease and therefore require secondary preventative measures, which will include statins to control their cholesterol.

Key points

- In severe obstetric hypertension, treatment is based on bringing the pregnancy to an end

- Perioperative hypertension is distinctly different from essential hypertension

- The treatment target in chronic kidney disease is 130/75 mmHg

- eGFR equals the percentage of remaining renal function

- Antithrombotic therapy in stroke should be delayed until the blood pressure is controlled

References

1. Roberts J, Gammill H. *Lancet* 2005;366(9490):961-962

2. Yorkshire Regional Severe Pre-Eclampsia Guidelines. Regional Advisory Panel: Tuffnell D, Walker J, Mason G, Lindow S, Lyons G, Russell I, Dresner M, Hawthorne L, Bickford Smith P, Jankowicz D. 4 March 2005

3. Dix P, Howell S. *Br J Anaesth* 2001;86(6):789-793

4. Prys-Roberts C. *Anaesthesia* 2001;56(6):505-510

Chapter **10**

When to give up

Learning objectives

In this chapter, we examine how to identify the patient on maximum tolerated therapy. We shall look at deciding who we should refer to specialists and when. In particular how should we manage the elderly patient? What do we do with the patient who cannot tolerate any medication or is never compliant?

Key words:

Maximum tolerated therapy

Side effects

Compliance

Adherence

Concordance

Resistance to therapy

Pseudohypertension

Referral

When to give up

In the real world we have to accept that we cannot successfully treat all patients. Some patients do not want to be treated; others cannot tolerate any form of medication; adherence can be variable; and many will not respond to the drugs we use. The UK's new General Medical Services (nGMS) Contract recognised this situation by offering the 'exception reporting' codes. One such code is the 'patient on maximum tolerated hypertensive therapy' code (Read code 8BL0). This sensible step indicates that we have tried to control the blood pressure but have failed. This introduces a new and important concept in the management of hypertension: namely, that there is an endpoint in trying to treat the patient. However, what is missing from the Contract is a definition of where that endpoint might be reached. Basically, it has been left to the discretion of individual doctors.

Using individual discretion usually leads to wide variations in practice. Therefore Dr Mark Davis and myself looked into producing some guidance to practitioners on behalf of the Primary Care Cardiovascular Society (PCCS). We discussed the matter with senior members of the British Hypertension Society, analysed current guidelines for references relevant to the issue, produced a draft set of guidelines and then further discussed the issues with doctors and nurses who were members of the PCCS. A full account of how we undertook this work is published in the *British Journal Of Cardiology*.[1] We arrived at the conclusions listed in *box 10.1*.

The PCCS maximal tolerated hypertension therapy guidelines: an explanation

It is important to have an evidence base to be able to justify your actions – hence the advice to follow the BHS or JBS Guidelines. The recommendation to have a clear written policy in your practice is a crucial point. The best policies are those that are produced locally based on national guidance. Adapting them to your practice, locality provider or primary care trust makes them more relevant and more likely to be adhered to.

Box 10.2 shows you how we adapted the maximum tolerated treatment guideline into a policy for my own practice. Note that we added our own points such as using three drugs in those aged over 80 years and listing

---

Box 10.1

The Primary Care Cardiovascular Society guidance on the coding of maximally tolerated blood pressure treatment:

- Follow the BHS or JBS Guidelines to justify your treatment policy

- Have a clear written policy in your practice as regards maximal treatment of blood pressure based on the BHS Guidelines

- If not contraindicated you should use four classes of drugs and if this fails to control your patients, or is not tolerated, you should consider referral to a specialist clinic

- In the patient aged over 80 years, if the standing systolic blood pressure falls by more than 20 mmHg, you should record the standing figures as your measure of control

- Patients aged over 80 years should be treated subject to individual clinical judgment, taking account of any comorbidity and their existing burden of drug use

- The patient's opinion should be taken into account and recorded before using the exception code

Ensure that you can justify your decisions to your Quality Outcome Framework (QOF) assessment panel and consider talking to panel members for guidance on these issues

---

beta-blocker contraindications. The former is not evidence based, but simply reflects our thinking on the matter. This is acceptable practice because we have written it down and received the approval of our local quality and outcomes (QOF) assessor. QOF assessors are local colleagues (doctors, nurses and lay people) who have been trained to assess and advise practices in terms of compliance with the nGMS Contract requirements. Initially they have been instructed to take a 'soft' approach to this work – in other words, help rather than punish practices that are struggling. The approach may harden in the future.

Box 10.2

Whitby Group Practice Policy on exception codes. 'Patient on maximum tolerated antihypertensive therapy' (8BL0):

- Always strive to control the patient's blood pressure; do not abuse exception codes

- If you do use exception codes you must justify their use in the patient's notes

- The patient must have a say in the use of exception codes and you should record their opinion

- Maximum therapy is achieved when four groups of drugs have been tried and are not tolerated, are contraindicated or failed to control blood pressure

- Maximum therapy is achieved in patients who are infirm or aged more than 80 years when three groups of drugs have been tried and either not tolerated, are contraindicated or failed to control blood pressure

- Consider referral of patients if control fails to meet audit target by more than 10/5 mmHg

- Beta-blocker contraindications include asthma, chronic obstructive pulmonary disease, heart block and the use of diltiazem

- Record the standing BP as the sitting BP if the patient has a postural drop of more than 20 mmHg

---

We recommended in the PCCS guidelines that 'if not contraindicated you should use four classes of drugs and if this fails to control your patients, or is not tolerated, you should consider referral to a specialist clinic'. The figure four was the consensus view of PCCS members and is not evidence based. However, it does fit in well with the BHS ABCD algorithm for the management of hypertension, as there is no fifth step in this.

Postural hypotension creates a real danger in elderly people of injury from falling, and balancing that risk against the peril of having untreated hypertension poses a substantial dilemma. We simply reiterated the advice contained in the BHS IV and the NICE Guidelines: namely, that 'in the patient aged over 80 years, if the standing systolic blood pressure falls by more than 20 mmHg you should record the standing figures as your measure of control'. This is one of the most important practical points and gets around the problem very easily. If the patient has postural hypotension, as defined by a systolic drop on standing of 20 mmHg, that does not mean they should be denied treatment for hypertension. It simply means you must judge the level of control by the standing instead of the sitting blood pressure. It is vital, however, that the blood pressure is recorded as a sitting rather than a standing measurement on your computer, as the latter is the parameter used for assessment under the nGMS Contract.

That patients aged over 80 years should be treated subject to individual clinical judgment, taking account of any comorbidity and their existing burden of drug use, is simply stating the obvious. The benefit of blood pressure lowering therapy in people over the age of 80 years has not yet been established. While those who reach 80 should continue on their treatment, no clear guidance can be given for those patients over that age who require initiation of therapy. We await the publication of the Hypertension in the Very Elderly Trial (HYVET) to help us answer this question.[2]

One of the most frequently made points by the PCCS members was that the patient's opinion should be taken into account. It is not acceptable that a doctor should make the decision to either continue or stop treatment in a patient without that patient's informed consent. Furthermore, a sensible doctor will record the reason why they feel justified in using a 'maximum treatment' code and indicate the patient's agreement.

Intolerance to medication

Intolerance can vary from mild side effects to total incapacity. It is very dependent on the attitude of the patient, and the more sceptical they are about the need for medication for an asymptomatic condition, the more likely they are to abandon the tablets.

Thiazide-like drugs (chlortalidone, indapamide) are sometimes better tolerated than thiazides (bendroflumethiazide, hydrochlorothiazide). ARBs are usually the best tolerated of all the various classes of antihypertensives.

The patient who can tolerate some drugs and is therefore receiving partial treatment should be reassured that they are receiving most of the benefits of treatment from the reduction they have achieved. If total control is going to be impossible then lifestyle interventions become even more important, and this needs to be stressed to the patient.

While it is common to have multiple drug intolerance it is rare not to be able to tolerate any medication whatsoever, but it happens. I would invariably refer such patients but the likelihood is that the specialist will also struggle to find a suitable drug and it is important that the patient does not expect too much.

These patients should be closely monitored and, if possible, all other risk factors for cardiovascular disease should be covered such as consideration of antiplatelet therapy, lipids and glycaemic control. Most importantly, the uncontrolled patient must not be abandoned; they still need 6-monthly checks.

Compliance, adherence and concordance

We are all well aware that whatever we say many patients will not take our advice on lifestyle and nor will they take the drugs we prescribe. Often this is obvious because we know they are not picking up the prescriptions, but equally it is not uncommon for a relative or friend to inform you that the patient is storing the tablets and not taking them.

In defining the term 'compliance' the *Concise Oxford Dictionary* uses words and phrases such as 'obedience', 'yield' and 'acquiescence to command'. Herein lies the problem. The doctor or nurse may be perceived as trying to get the patient to bend to their wishes; it might be an issue about control. It might be that the patient is getting side effects, such as impotence, and is simply too embarrassed to tell the doctor because they do not want to discuss them, or they are simply afraid of letting down somebody for whom

---

Box 10.3

Factors in poor compliance:

- Patient perception
- Side effects
- Misunderstanding
- Guilt
- Embarrassment
- Anxiety
- Low IQ
- Poverty
- Alcoholism
- Prescription charges
- Carer collusion

Factors in improved compliance:

- Full explanation
- Empowerment
- Trust
- Concordance/agreement
- Side effect warnings
- Once-daily dosing
- Fixed-dose combinations
- Prepayment certificates
- Computer records
- Home BP monitors

---

they have a lot of respect. Sometimes it is due to a simple misunderstanding – some patients do not realise they have to keep taking the tablets to continue to benefit. Certain types of patient are more likely to fail to comply, such as those of low IQ, low socioeconomic standing, alcoholics and the anxious. The fact that many have to pay a prescription charge may be a factor, and it is very important that the patient is made aware of the savings that can be made by using the prepayment method. Incidentally, I feel it is very unfair that people with hypertension are excluded from free prescriptions while diabetic patients are included, and I find it very hard to understand the justification behind this policy.

Computerised prescribing has been of huge assistance in spotting the patient who does not ask for repeat prescriptions. You could go to great lengths to spot non-adherence, such as the methods used in some pharmaceutical trials – for example, urine or serum assays of the drug or using electronic pill dispensers that record each access. However, I feel that if you exhibit this level of mistrust of the patient you are unlikely to build much of a relationship to enhance compliance.

The key to improving adherence is in achieving **concordance** (harmonious agreement) or, in other words, empowering the patient. The very word 'compliance' is probably not appropriate because it suggests that the doctor is expecting the patient to bend to his or her will. 'Adherence' (to stick to, follow, support) is a more accurate reflection of what we mean in that it implies that the patient is sticking to their medication, following advice and supporting the doctor's endeavours. But what we really need is **concordance** or the mutual agreement of doctor and patient on a plan of action that is part of a contract. Ask the patient if they are happy to go along with treatment, warn them of side effects in advance, make it clear that if they do not consent it is their choice, and explain that the treatment is for their sake and not yours – although the advent of nGMS inducement payments might make it more difficult to be convincing about this! Once-daily dosing and fixed-dose combinations make it more simple to take medication and can be of psychological assistance to the patient. Home monitoring of blood pressure may help in some cases.

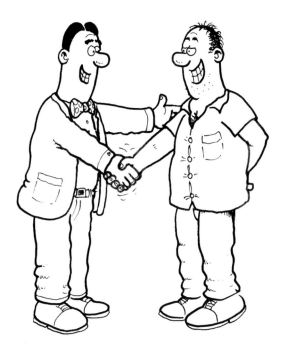

Concordance is the mutual agreement of doctor and patient on a plan of action

Resistance to therapy

There are patients who tolerate their therapy but, despite taking four or even five drugs at maximum doses, remain uncontrolled. This may be because of secondary hypertension, particularly where there is a mechanism requiring high blood pressure to maintain function, such as in stenosis of arteries. Elderly patients may have irreversible arteriosclerosis, which will be particularly unresponsive to attempts at vasodilatation. This may reflect a compensatory adaptation to longstanding untreated hypertension. Your drugs may be interacting with other drugs, and in particular the patient might have an alcohol problem. Excess salt intake will counteract the effects of ACE inhibitors. But it may simply come back down to non-adherence.

Box 10.4

Reasons for resistance to therapy:

- Secondary hypertension
  - Conn's syndrome
  - primary aldosteronism
  - coarctation of aorta
  - aortic stenosis
  - renal artery stenosis
- Atherosclerosis in the elderly
  - pseudohypertension
- Concomitant therapy
  - steroids
  - NSAIDs
  - alcohol
- Excess salt intake
- Non-adherence

Pseudohypertension is a term used by the American Heart Association (AHA) to describe a condition where the peripheral arteries of very elderly patients become so stiff that they cannot be compressed by the cuff without excess pressure being applied. This gives a falsely elevated blood pressure that cannot respond to treatment. It should be suspected if the brachial or radial arteries are still palpable in a fully inflated cuff (Osler's sign). Patients with this condition are few in number and should not be classified as having hypertension.[3]

Deciding when to refer

The BHS IV Guidelines recommend that patients should be referred to a specialist service in cases of multiple drug intolerance, multiple drug contraindications, persistent non-adherence, persistent non-compliance (note that the BHS uses both phrases) and resistance to three or more drugs. I would in fact take issue with this advice. First, many areas do not have specialist clinics and rely on referral to hospital physicians or cardiologists who may not have any particular interest or training in the treatment of hypertension. Second, the BHS's ABCD table gives clear advice on how to treat people resistant to three drugs, and I feel the primary care physician should follow that advice before referral. Third, it entirely escapes me how the specialist is going to enforce compliance. When I asked Dr Phil Avery, full-time cardiologist and part-time musician, why he felt the patient was more likely to comply with his treatment than mine, he told me that it was obviously because he wore a white coat! But my fourth objection is the clincher. If all the primary care physicians in the UK complied with this advice the hospital clinics would be overrun and the very valuable work they are already providing would suffer.

Ultimately the GP will use discretion and common sense when deciding to refer. Very young patients, the pregnant patient and those with complicated comorbidity such as renal disease or possible secondary hypertension will take precedence. In the Whitby Group Practice Policy *(see box 10.2)* we make the point that the doctor should 'consider referral of patients if control fails to meet audit target by more than 10/5 mmHg'. The rationale here is that, if a patient is taking four drugs and has reached a blood pressure of say 151/91 mmHg, it is unlikely that a specialist will want to become involved just to satisfy the need for the GP to hit a payment target. But at 161/96 mmHg the specialist is more likely to feel it is an appropriate referral.

GPs will vary in terms of confidence and competence in this subject but, ultimately, referral may have more to do with liability and where the 'buck stops' than with looking for a definitive treatment for the patient.

Who do you refer to? In large cities there are usually hypertension clinics run by experts in clinical therapeutics, epidemiology, cardiology or renal medicine. In small district general hospitals this may not be the case. Some renal physicians will have a special interest and agree to see non-renal disease patients, but often referral is to the local cardiologist who may not have any formal training in hypertension. Hopefully, this will change in future. The creation of a new field of 'vascular specialists' is in the planning stages. These doctors' projected areas of expertise would encompass hypertension, lipids, diabetes, cardiology, peripheral vascular disease, renal medicine and stroke. They sound a bit like GPs to me!

Key points

- Enter a written justification of your use of the 'maximally tolerated blood pressure treatment' code in the patient's notes

- In patients aged over 80 years, if the standing systolic blood pressure falls by more than 20 mmHg, you should record the standing figures as your measure of control

- The patient who has uncontrolled blood pressure will still benefit from lifestyle advice and consideration for antiplatelet, lipid control and antiglycaemic therapy.

- Compliance is best achieved through concordance

References

1. McCormack T, Davis M. *Br J Cardiol* 2005;12:156-160

2. Bulpitt CJ, Fletcher A, Beckett NS et al. *Drugs Aging* 2001;18:151-164

3. Pickering TG, Hall JE, Appel LJ. *J Clin Hypertens* 2005;7(2):102-109

Chapter **11**

Case histories

Five case histories are used to illustrate some of the points made in the book. They are highly anonymised accounts of the experiences of real patients, and all names have been changed.

A novel birthday present

Mike is a slim, 60-year-old taxi driver who looks younger than his age. Occasionally he needs creams for his dermatitis but otherwise he is a stranger to us at the surgery. He recently received a private health check as a birthday present from his family. Just the thing to make you feel your age!

Mike arrived at my surgery after the check with the news that there was something wrong with his blood pressure and cholesterol, which were 150/90 mmHg and 6.4 mmol/l, respectively. Initially I thought this was all a bit over the top because the figures were not too bad in someone with no pre-existing cardiovascular disease or diabetes, but when I looked at all the facts things were very different. The report he had been given after the health check detailed his high-density lipoprotein cholesterol (HDL-C) as 1.3 mmol/l and this gave him a total cholesterol (TC):HDL ratio of 4.9 mmol/l. I repeated his blood pressure and the average of two resting measurements was 155/85 mmHg. His only other risk factor was that of having a lifelong smoking habit of 15 cigarettes a day.

The private clinic had used the old Joint British Society (JBS) Guidelines risk calculator and arrived at a surprisingly high score of 25% coronary heart disease (CHD) risk over 10 years, which when projected to age 69 years equalled a risk of 31%. I rechecked this with the new JBS 2 risk calculator, which gave Mike a 34% absolute risk of suffering a cardiovascular (CVD) event in the next decade and rose to a frightening 45% when calculated to the age point 69 years. Using the computer risk calculator I was also able to demonstrate to Mike that his risk relative to his peer group was a staggering 82 out of 100. I could also show him that if he stopped smoking his relative risk fell to 42; if we brought his systolic blood pressure down to the target of 140 mmHg the relative risk went further down to 33; and that if we achieved the total cholesterol target of 4.0 mmol/l it dropped to an impressive 2.

Without his family paying for a private check we would not have realised the severity of Mike's risk, and he would have been deprived the low-dose aspirin, statin and blood pressure treatment he clearly warranted. Despite this stark lesson I cannot promise to provide this sort of comprehensive screening for everyone on our list simply because we do not have the resources. Hence we have to target the very highest risk patients, namely those with known moderate to severe hypertension and the obese – of course, Mike was not a member of either of those groups! Diabetics are treated as a separate case under the new guidelines.

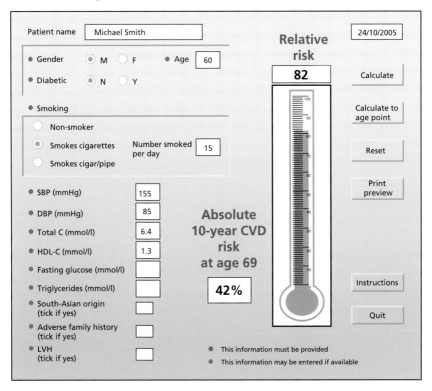

Mike's absolute and relative risk of coronary heart disease

Lessons learnt here

Apparently healthy patients can be at high risk of cardiovascular disease. Smoking and low HDL are especially influential risk factors. The new JBS 2 risk tables indicate overall cardiovascular risk, and there is an age correction that has a marked effect for some individuals.

She makes me laugh

Box 11.1

Patient's hypertension uncontrolled despite taking:

- Bendroflumethiazide 2.5 mg

- Atenolol 100 mg

- Nifedipine LA 40 mg

- Doxazosin 8 mg

- Moxonidine 200 mg tds

Marion is a 60-year-old overweight lady with a great sense of humour who smokes 30 cigarettes a day. She has a past history of mild COPD, hiatus hernia, cholecystitis and sciatica. Her lifestyle is responsible for most of her ill health but she is resistant to change on a philosophical basis. Seven years ago she suffered a small right-sided hemiplegia with 4/5th weakness that resolved fully after 2 days – a subsequent CAT scan was reported as normal. This episode revealed an underlying severe hypertension with blood pressures ranging from 176/92 to 230/104 mmHg. She was prescribed bendroflumethiazide, then atenolol (despite her COPD), then nifedipine, followed by an ACE inhibitor that she could not tolerate due to dizziness, then a sartan, which caused the same side effect, and eventually doxazosin too. Despite good compliance with maximum doses of the four drugs that she was able to tolerate, her blood pressure still ranged from 160/75 to 176/82 mmHg. Moxonidine 200 mg three times daily was added with very little effect. It was then noted on a routine blood test that her potassium was 2.5 mmol/l and, in fact, looking back over the 2 years since her stroke it had never been higher than 3.1 mmol/l. The penny dropped! She was an uncontrolled hypertensive with a hypokalaemia, which at her age could not be explained by taking the bendroflumethiazide alone. She was most likely suffering from primary aldosteronism, or maybe even Conn's syndrome.

Her care was already being shared with the local cardiologists in view of the difficulties we were having controlling her blood pressure. Because of the low potassium we stopped her thiazide, and she was admitted for investigation as an urgent case. On admission she was jointly cared for by the cardiology and biochemistry consultants. She had all her medication stopped and was placed on enforced bedrest with frequent blood pressure monitoring. Her blood pressure did rise but not by very much. Ambulatory and supine aldosterone levels were within the normal range, and renin levels were also normal, throughout her stay. A non-spiral CAT scan of abdomen revealed no tumour of the adrenal gland. Despite these results it was felt that it would be prudent to try a small dose of spironolactone 25 mg on this lady as well as resuming all her pre-admission drugs, apart from bendroflumethiazide. I saw her 3 weeks after discharge and her blood pressure was a jaw-dropping 144/72 mmHg; 2 weeks later she was at 137/66 mmHg. She now takes spironolactone 25 mg, verapamil 120 mg bd, doxazosin 8 mg, simvastatin 40 mg, aspirin 75 mg and her inhalers. She remains well controlled but feels very flat as a result of all her drugs. She still smokes, remains very overweight, enjoys the perk of free food at her place of employment and makes me cry with laughter every time I see her.

Lessons learnt here

Marion was probably suffering from primary aldosteronism, but this was not Conn's syndrome because she did not have an adrenal tumour. Investigating these conditions is very difficult - and in this case disproved the diagnosis. However a trial of spironolactone was so successful it cast doubt on the sensitivity of Marion's investigations. Diagnosis of primary aldosteronism and Conn's syndrome is now based on renin:aldosterone ratios, and it is no longer necessary to stop all medication.

This case had a great influence on my attitude to Conn's syndrome and aldosteronism, and I have become a keen advocate of the use of spironolactone in hypertension as well as heart failure. The caveat to that enthusiasm is that spironolactone must be used with great care. Regular monitoring of electrolytes is required and, in particular, the patient must be warned to temporally stop the medication if they have a diarrhoea.

Too many Mars bars

Bernard was 45 years old when he had his myocardial infarction. Thanks to his schizophrenia he was neglecting himself and living in squalid conditions. It was during his hospital stay that he was noted to have essential hypertension. His diet appeared to consist mainly of Mars bars and his BMI was 34 kg/m^2. A year after his heart attack we also discovered that he had diabetes mellitus. It was very difficult to get Bernard to take his medication, and his blood pressure and diabetes were therefore uncontrolled. He was also suffering from angina. Everyone involved in his care agreed that it was only a matter of time before he suffered another event and that he was unlikely to enjoy a long life. That was 12 years ago.

Because of the seemingly impossible task of being able to help Bernard, a very enterprising psychiatric social worker organised a Guardianship Order under Section 7 of the Mental Health Act. Bernard was initially a reluctant participant in this but he now realises how much he has benefited from the order. This allowed social services to take over his finances, establish a supervised residence for him and gain daily access to administer his medication, which is delivered weekly in a blister pack. All of this is expensive, but in Bernard's case it is lifesaving. Social services asked if he could have all his medication once daily to reduce visits and keep expenses down. His current medication is listed in *box 11.2*. He really should be taking insulin, but we felt this posed too much of a risk because of his unsupervised periods and, of course, would require a daily visit from a district nurse as well as the care worker.

Our approach has been a success in terms of maintaining both Bernard's health and his relative independence. Unfortunately he still likes his Mars bars, but that is his choice and there is little we can do about it.

Box 11.2

Bernard's current medication:

- Aspirin 75 mg
- Bisoprolol 10 mg
- Isosorbide mononitrate SR 60 mg
- Simvastatin 40 mg
- Bendroflumethiazide 2.5 mg
- Angiotensin receptor blocker (maximum dose)
- Gliclazide MR
- Thiazolidinedione (glitazone)
- Metformin 1 g
- Risperidone 2 mg

Lessons learnt here

Just because the patient puts barriers in the way of their treatment does not mean they cannot be overcome. Psychosocially disadvantaged patients are most likely to be non-compliant with their medication. The measures employed here are somewhat extreme and could not be used for all patients with adherence problems. There has to be some element of compromise - such as the once-daily medication, lack of insulin and Mars bars arrangements here - and that is part of the agreement required to empower the patient.

You can't win them all

Tommy was a 63-year-old gardener with no particularly exciting past medical history who came to the surgery complaining of shortness of breath with moderate exertion. He was also describing orthopnoea and, on examination, he had a tachycardia with gallop rhythm and no murmur. His blood pressure was 190/110 mmHg. An electrocardiogram showed evidence of non-specific ischaemia changes. This very much looked like a case of heart failure secondary to either hypertension or ischaemia and so I prescribed furosemide 80 mg and advised him to stop smoking immediately, which he did.

I saw him again the following week. I had ordered a chest X-ray, which was reported as 'heart size normal and lungs clear'. He had improved a little with the furosemide and his blood pressure was now 192/118 mmHg. I decided to organise an open access echocardiogram but, as his blood pressure was still very high and heart failure was the most likely cause, I decided to initiate lisinopril 2.5 mg while we awaited the investigation. He returned the next week and his blood pressure was now 170/96 mmHg and his creatinine 159 µmol/l, which was slightly higher than his pre-prescription reading of 147 µmol/l. I decided to press on with controlling his blood pressure and increased the dose of lisinopril to 5 mg daily. Two weeks later his blood pressure was 146/88 mmHg but his creatinine had risen to 174 µmol/l. He reported feeling much better so I decided to keep him on the 5 mg dose of the ACE inhibitor and repeat his creatinine in another 2 weeks time.

We have a very good local echocardiography service, so when Tommy returned I had both the echo report and his latest renal function results. The echo report stated 'reasonable left ventricular function with an ejection fraction of 57%, minor mitral regurgitation, tricuspid valve normal and a slightly thickened aortic valve. Pressure gradient 14 mmHg.' His serum creatinine was now 204 µmol/l. I was getting a little concerned that things were 'not right' here. The test results did not really fit in with heart failure and the deterioration in renal function was worrying despite the fact that Tommy felt a lot better. I reduced the lisinopril to 2.5 mg and ordered an urgent renal ultrasound to look for evidence of renal artery stenosis. He did not have any symptoms of peripheral arterial disease and he had reasonable foot pulses.

The ultrasound report was quite shocking. It showed 'a large aortic aneurysm extending 13 cms from the bifurcation. It was not possible to visualise the renal arteries. Maximum AP diameter 6.5 cms, maximum transverse diameter 7.3 cms. Right kidney small 6.3 cms and showing cortical thinning. Liver slightly enlarged but no other abnormality noted.'

Tommy was seen very quickly by the local vascular surgeons and within 2 months he had undergone a repair of his infra-renal aortic aneurysm. Unfortunately he went into renal failure postoperatively and had to go on dialysis. Three months after his operation he died of a pulmonary embolus.

Lessons learnt here

We often have to start treatment on a hunch. The only part of the diagnosis that I got right here was that he was hypertensive, and controlling that was important. ACE inhibitors are useful drugs but monitoring renal function in patients taking them is vital, especially in the early stages of therapy. If the creatinine does not rise by much, continue therapy with caution. When the creatinine starts to climb rapidly reduce the dose, rather than stop the drug. Sudden curtailment of an ACE inhibitor can have a catastrophic effect.

Renal artery stenosis will give you a small kidney, and clearly there was some involvement already. Repairs of aneurysms near the renal artery carry the worst prognosis. With hindsight, although he probably would have died suddenly at some point, Tommy would have been better off left untreated, but of course I had no way of knowing that.

I'm happy just as I am

Dick is a 49-year-old, happy-go-lucky carpet salesman with an ever present smile. Unfortunately, despite his good cheer, he was diagnosed as having essential hypertension 9 years ago. He also smokes 60 cigarettes a day and with a TC of 6.2 mmol/l and a HDL-C of 1.02 mmol/l, giving a ratio of 6.08, he needs more than just blood pressure control. The problem is that, while Dick has been made aware that he has three major risk factors for cardiovascular disease, it is not in his nature to succumb to any real concern. He did not get the label of 'Mr Happy' by being a worrier.

He rarely comes to see me and, were it not for his occasional migraine and his need to attend for medication reviews to stock up with sumatriptan, I don't think he would ever come. He is obviously embarrassed about his smoking habit and assumes I am going to 'tell him off' each time we meet, even though I never have.

Initially I prescribed atenolol for his blood pressure of 172/102 mmHg because of his age and in the hope it might help his migraine.

Having asked him to return in 2 weeks, I next saw him a year later when he had run out of sumatriptan! Because he could not stand the fatigue elicited by the atenolol he had stopped it as soon as his supply was exhausted. He was amazed that his blood pressure was now 176/100 mmHg despite not taking any medication for 11 months. I prescribed lisinopril, starting at 5 mg daily, and explained in great detail his need to keep taking the tablets, undergo blood tests, return for uptitration, etc.

He did return for his blood test but not for the uptitration. The tablets were available on repeat prescription in an attempt to help him comply with treatment - unlike his sumatriptan, which I was using as a carrot. When I saw him again, 6 months later, he had collected two repeat prescriptions of lisinopril (one 2 weeks before his appointment with me). There was a slight reduction in his BP to 166/98 mmHg. I increased the dose of lisinopril to 10 mg and again emphasised the need for better adherence to the medication plan. At his next overdue visit he told me his 'smokers cough' became much worse during the months he took his tablets! Because of his ACE inhibitor cough I prescribed a sartan. This was well tolerated, and he was clearly taking the tablets more days than not, because at his next visit his blood pressure had come down to a reasonable 154/98 mmHg. But as he was still not at target, I did something I do not usually do: I prescribed a fixed-dose combination of the same sartan with a thiazide diuretic.

At the next behind-schedule meeting, Dick informed me that a good friend of his had had a stroke. This was lucky for Dick, if not for the friend, as it seemed to have done the trick with his compliance – now his blood pressure was a stunning 135/79 mmHg. I thought I would take advantage of his sudden conversion to conformity and prescribed simvastatin 40 mg for his raised cholesterol.

At our most recent meeting he informed me that he had stopped the hypertension treatment while taking the statin, as he did not believe in overdoing the pills. He further informed me that he had then stopped the statin after 2 weeks due to myalgia and gone back to the sartan and thiazide combination. He was very proud of having cut down his smoking habit to only 20 a day! I might claim a partial victory perhaps?

Lessons learned here

Patients are more likely to comply with medication regimens that give them symptomatic relief such as proton pump inhibitors and migraine treatments. You might be able to use this to encourage visits. Recent evidence has come to light linking migraines with atrial septal defects[1] and therefore an echocardiogram might have been indicated here.

Computer records allow us to track how many prescriptions are picked up. It is important to persevere, even if the patient is not a willing subject, and to accept compromise. The number of tablets prescribed is an issue and, psychologically, patients may be happier with increased use of fixed-dose combinations.

Reference

1. Wilmshurst PT, Pearson MJ, Nightingale S et al. *Heart* 2004; 90:1315-1320

Appendix 1

Home blood pressure monitoring

Date of test	15-8-05

Name	Amy Body
Date of birth	29-2-53
Computer number	987653

	Systolic BP (top number)	Diastolic BP (bottom number)	Pulse
Initial clinic BP	180	88	72

Home readings

Day 1 before 10 am	164	88	63
Day 1 between 10 am and 4 pm	140	68	59
Day 1 between 4 pm and 8 pm	133	76	60
Day 1 after 8 pm	161	83	52
Day 2 before 10 am	137	68	62
Day 2 between 10 am and 4 pm	122	60	57
Day 2 between 4 pm and 8 pm	120	73	73
Day 2 after 8 pm	156	87	52
TOTAL of all home readings	1133	603	
DIVIDE by 8	142	75	
ADD	10	5	
Corrected home blood pressure	152	80	

Appendix 2

Whitby Group Practice Hypertension Protocol 2005

Blood pressure measurement

- Use the left arm and the correct cuff size

- The lowest reading after sitting for 10 minutes is the most accurate

- Home measurements must be adjusted by adding 10/5 mmHg

- In the elderly, if standing systolic drops by >20 mmHg, record the standing BP as the sitting measurement

Diagnostic criteria

- If normal, recheck in 5 years

- Take four readings on four separate occasions if abnormal

- If moderate, at least 2 weeks apart

- If severe, at least 1 day apart

- If average is normal/mild after four readings recheck in 1 year

- At least one check by nurse, one by doctor

- Labile hypertension should be treated

- Do not code as essential hypertension unless treatment is indicated

Definition of moderate hypertension

(BHS guidelines state that mild hypertension alone does not need medication)

- Systolic BP 160 mmHg or more

- Diastolic BP 100 mmHg or more

- Diastolic BP >90 mmHg + target organ damage

- Treat if either systolic or diastolic raised

- Age is irrelevant (absolute risk greatest in elderly)

- Severe is 180/110 mmHg or more

Target organ damage

- Left ventricular hypertrophy
  (sum of R & S >37 mm plus inverted T in V5 & V6)

- Heart failure

- Renal impairment

- Ischaemic heart disease

- Cerebrovascular disease

- Peripheral vascular disease

- Retinal changes

New GMS Contract audit targets

- Smoking status and advice offered every 15 months

- *BP indicator 5.* BP 150/90 mmHg or less: 57 points (70%)
  measured every 9 months

- *CHD indicator 6.* BP 150/90 mmHg or less: 19 points (70%)
  measured every 15 months

- *Stroke indicator 6.* BP 150/90 mmHg or less: 5 points (70%)
  measured every 15 months

- *Diabetes indicator 12.* BP 145/85 mmHg or less: 18 points (60%)
  measured every 15 months

White coat hypertension

- Home BP monitor readings must be equated to clinic reading
  – add 10 mmHg to systolic and 5 mmHg to diastolic

- White coat hypertension may mask hypertension

- Need annual home BP checks

Patient assessment

- Smoker?

- Excess alcohol?

- Drugs (pill/steroids)?

- FH of cardiovascular disease under 65 years in female or 55 years in male?

- Weight

- CVS

- Fundi (optional)

Investigation

- Urinalysis for protein

- FBC

- U&Es

- Random blood glucose

- LFTs

- Gamma GT

- Uric acid

- ECG

- Non-fasting total cholesterol and HDL (follow lipid protocol)

Consider

- Chest X-ray (LVH)

- Ultrasound scan of abdomen (arterial disease, raised creatinine)

- Conn's syndrome/primary aldosteronism – hypokalaemia, alkalosis, sodium slightly raised

- Phaechromocytoma – very rare; vanillymandelic acid (young, acute anxiety attacks)

Non-drug treatment

- Stop smoking

- Avoid saturated fats: <1 g/100 g

- Lose weight: 10% or 10 kg

- Take regular exercise: 30 minutes' walking on five occasions a week

- Do not add salt to food

- Reduce alcohol intake

Medication

- Tailored to individual needs/pre-existing pathology

- Three drugs often required for control: 60% of patients need two drugs

- Use BHS ABCD tables

- In monotherapy use maximum doses

- In combination therapy use optimal doses

Group	First choice	Second choice
Diuretic	Bendroflumethazide 2.5 mg	Indapamide

especially: elderly, systolic hypertension
side effects: impotence, diabetes, gout, low K+

Beta-blocker	Metoprolol	Bisoprolol

especially: IHD
side effects: asthma, heart failure, peripheral vascular disease, heart block, impotence

Angiotensin blockade	Lisinopril	Specific sartan

contraindications: pregnancy
side effects: renal failure. Lisinopril only; cough, severe allergy

Ca++ antagonist	Felodipine	Diltiazem

especially: peripheral vascular disease, angina.
side effects: flushing, headache, swollen ankles, indigestion

Fourth line	Spironolactone	Doxazosin

Follow-up and nurses' clinic

• Review fortnightly until controlled

• When controlled enter nurse review in 6 months and medication review 12 months

• Nurse review includes:

  – urinalysis every time

- cholesterol check if indicated

- *U&Es if on diuretic, ACE inhibitor or renal disease*

• Alternate doctor/nurse or nurse practitioner reviews every 6 months

• Yearly review if treatment stopped or white coat hypertension

• If not controlled refer to doctor

Over 80 years

• If postural drop of 20 mmHg systolic then enter the standing BP (lower figure) as the sitting BP

• No more than three drugs

• Stop drugs if not tolerated

Exception codes - Whitby Group Practice Policy

'Patient on maximum tolerated anti-hypertensive therapy' (8BL0)
'Beta-blockers contraindicated' (8I26)

• Always strive to control the patient's blood pressure; do not abuse exception codes

• If you do use exception codes you must justify their use in the patient's notes

• The patient must have a say in the use of exception codes and you should record their opinion

• Maximum therapy is achieved when four groups of drugs have been tried and either not tolerated, are contraindicated or failed to control blood pressure

• Maximum therapy is achieved in patients who are infirm or aged more than 80 years when three groups of drugs have been tried and either not tolerated, are contraindicated or failed to control blood pressure

- Consider referral of patients if control fails to meet audit target by more than 10/5 mmHg

- Beta-blocker contraindications include asthma, chronic obstructive pulmonary disease, heart block and the use of diltiazem

- Record the standing BP as the sitting BP if the patient has a postural drop of more than 20 mmHg

Appendix 3

Whitby Group Practice Lipids Protocol 2006

Is there a reason to carry out a cholesterol test?

Secondary prevention

All patients with history of:

- Myocardial infarction

- Angina

- CABG or angioplasty

- Peripheral vascular disease (also require fasting triglycerides once, treat if >5.0 mmol/l)

- CVA

- Diabetes

Treat if average total cholesterol of 5.0 mmol/l or above

Initiate treatment in over-80's at patient's discretion

Suspected primary lipid disorder

Family history of;

- Familial hyperlipidaemia or

- First-line relative (father, mother, brother, sister) IHD <55 ♂ ,<65 ♀

- Tendon xanthoma, xanthelasma, arcus senilis (refer to doctor)

Primary prevention

Test if age >40 years and

- Hypertensive

- BMI >30 kg/m² or waist measurement >102 cm, 88 cm

Treat lipids and BP if they have risk of CVD ≥20%/10 years (CHD >15%)

JBS risk table equivalents/10 years

Coronary heart disease (CHD) risk = cardiovascular disease (CVD) risk

Existing risk calculator vs new risk calculator

CHD 15% = CVD 20%

CHD 22% = CVD 30%

CHD 30% = CVD 40%

Treat lipids if they have total cholesterol (TC):HDL ratio ≥6.0, irrespective of risk assessment

Which tests?

Secondary prevention

- Initially do non-fasting TC, TSH, LFTs, U&Es and glucose and treat on those results

- Follow-up should be with random TC and LFTs at 3 months then yearly when controlled (at 1 month with rosuvastatin)

Suspected primary lipid disorder

- Initially do non-fasting TC, HDL-C and glucose

- If cholesterol >9.0 mmol/l or TC:HDL ratio >6.0 do fasting cholesterol, HDL, triglycerides, TSH, LFTs, U&Es and glucose

Primary prevention

- Initially do non-fasting TC, HDL-C, TSH, LFTs, U&Es and glucose and treat on result

- Follow-up as with secondary prevention

Treatment

- All patients must be advised on correct diet

- Initially prescribe simvastatin 20 mg nocte for 1 month and then simvastatin 40 mg

After 3 months retest cholesterol & LFTs. If target level not achieved:

- Prescribe two simvastatin 40 mg (nocte)

  - not if elderly or on drugs that interact (see list below)

If target level not achieved after 1 month

- Prescribe powerful statin X mg (any time of day)

If target level not achieved after 1 month

- Prescribe powerful statin 2X mg (any time of day)

If target level not achieved after further 1 month

- Prescribe simvastatin 40 mg/ezetimibe 10 mg nocte

If target level not achieved after further 1 month

- Prescribe powerful statin 2X mg and ezetimibe 10 mg (any time of day)

If target level not achieved after further 1 month

- Refer to specialist and notify TM

If AST/ALT x3 upper limit of normal, stop statin

Check CK if patient complains of myalgia

- if CK x5 upper limit of normal, recheck after 1 week; if same stop statin

- if CK x10 upper limit of normal stop statin

After reaching target level you should retest cholesterol yearly and also perform LFTs

Fasting triglycerides are required in peripheral vascular disease or familial cases.

- if above 5.0 mmol/l seek advice regarding treatment

Bezafibrate or fenofibrate are alternative drugs if statins are not tolerated

Secondary causes of hyperlipidaemia

High cholesterol

- Hypothyroidism

- Biliary obstruction

- Nephrotic syndrome

- Thiazide diuretics

- Steroids

- Contraceptive pill

High triglycerides

- Diabetes

- Alcohol abuse

- Chronic renal failure

- Bulimia

Drug interactions with statins

Interactions are more likely in renal impairment, liver disease, old age, low body weight and following major surgery. Pravastatin (a weak statin) is less likely to react with these drugs:

- Fibrates, gemfibrozil, nicotinic acid

- Antiviral 'avirs' in HIV treatment doses

- 'Azoles' antifungals

- Coumarins, warfarin

- Ciclosporin

- Digoxin, amiodarone

- Erythromycin, clarithromycin, fucidin
  (stop statin temporarily while taking these)

- Protease inhibitors, diltiazem, verapamil, antacids

- Grapefruit juice, Chinese red rice

Exception codes - Whitby Group Practice Policy

'Patient on maximum tolerated lipid lowering therapy' (8BL1)

'Statin contraindicated' (8I27)

'Statin declined' (8I3C)

- Always strive to control the patients' cholesterol; do not abuse exception codes

- If you do use exception codes you must justify their use in the patient's notes

- The patient must have a say in the use of exception codes and you should record their opinion

- Maximum therapy is achieved when the steps in the protocol have been tried and are not tolerated, are contraindicated or failed to control cholesterol

- There is no evidence that patients over 80 years benefit from having lipid therapy initiated, but there is evidence that those already on therapy do benefit

- Consider referral of patients if they have familial hypercholesterolaemia

- Statin contraindications include renal failure, liver disease and many drugs which interact with these compounds (see list, above)

Further reading

1. Beevers G, Lip GYH, O'Brien E. *ABC of hypertension*, 4th ed. London: BMJ Books, 2001.

2. Brady A, Petrie J. *New perspectives on hypertension.* Weybridge, UK: Merit Publishing International, 2003.

3. Kimpson P, Howell S. *The physiology of the control of blood pressure and antihypertensive drugs.* London: Royal College of Anaesthetists, Bulletin 25, May 2004.

Index